Alzheimer Discourse:
Some Sociolinguistic Dimensions

LEA's Communication Series
Jennings Bryant/Dolf Zillmann, General Editors

Selected titles in Language and Communication (Donald Ellis, Advisory Editor) include:

Ramanathan • Alzheimer Discourse: Some Sociolinguistic Dimensions
Haslet/Samter • Children Communicating: The First Five Years
Campbell • Coherence, Continuity, and Cohesion: Theoretical Foundations
    for Document Design
Ellis • From Language to Communication
Sigman • Consequentiality of Communication
Tracy • Understanding Face-to-Face Interactions

For a complete list of other titles in LEA's Communication Series, please contact Lawrence Erlbaum Associates, Publishers.

Alzheimer Discourse:
Some Sociolinguistic Dimensions

Vai Ramanathan
University of Alabama

LAWRENCE ERLBAUM ASSOCIATES, PUBLISHERS
1997   Mahwah, New Jersey   London

Copyright © 1997 by Lawrence Erlbaum Associates, Inc.
All rights reserved. No part of the book may be reproduced in any form, by photostat, microform, retrieval system, or any other means without the prior written consent of the publisher.

Lawrence Erlbaum Associates, Inc., Publishers
10 Industrial Avenue
Mahwah, NJ 07430

Cover design by Mairav Salomon-Dekel

Library of Congress Cataloging-in-Publication Data

Ramanathan, Vai
    Alzheimer discourse : some sociolinguistic dimensions / Vai Ramanathan
        p. cm
    Includes bibliographical references and index
    ISBN 0-8058-2354-9 (cloth : alk. paper). — ISBN 0-8058-2355-7 (pbk. : alk. paper)
    1. Alzheimer's disease—Patients—Language. 2. Sociolinguistics. I. Title.
RC523.R35   1997
616.8'31—dc21   96–48217
                                                            CIP

Books published by Lawrence Erlbaum Associates are printed on acid-free paper, and their bindings are chosen for strength and durability.

Printed in the United States of America

10 9 8 7 6 5 4 3 2 1

For Aasha
My joy, my peace

Contents

	Acknowledgments	ix
1	Introduction	1
2	Theoretical Framework	11
3	Wellformedness in Alzheimer Interactions: Continuity Elements	30
4	Narrative and Interactive Illformedness in Alzheimer Talk	53
5	Repair as a Discontinuity Element: Examining Tina's Talk With N	71
6	A Schematic Understanding of Repetition in an AD Life Story	89
7	Some Implications and Conclusions	116
	References	127
	Author Index	133
	Subject Index	136

Acknowledgments

This book argues that almost everything we say depends, to a large extent, on whom or what we are interacting with, that social factors influence not only what we say, but the fluency and ease with which we say it as well. Thus, to acknowledge the contribution of some people who made this book happen is to thank them in a small way not only for shaping my ideas and views but also for enabling me to speak.

My professors at the University of Southern California—Elaine Anderson, Ed Finegan, James Gee, Robert Kaplan, Elinor Ochs—introduced me to the multifaceted prism that linguistics is and taught me in their individual ways that language use is always and everywhere social. James Gee, my mentor, told me on several occasions that his research was interest on the capital *his* mentors had given him; I think I know now what he meant. I like to think that the research represented in this book is interest gained on the time and effort he spent in reading several drafts and providing valuable feedback. His views about discourse analysis—its moral function and humanistic value—have influenced me enormously.

Although Robert Kaplan has little direct connection to Alzheimer discourse, his friendship and support in almost every other area of my life have been tremendous. Our overlapping research interests and e-mail discussions on issues in second language literacy have in some strange way percolated down to the analysis presented here. His foresight, clarity, and bird's-eye view of all matters linguistic are things from which I have benefited immensely. I have adopted him as my godparent whether he likes it or not.

I need to thank several other people as well. It was a pleasure to work with Don Ellis, the series editor, whose views and research on discourse I find stimulating. I especially appreciate his easygoing manner and the latitude he allowed me throughout this project. Heidi Hamilton's feedback on some of my writing and her general enthusiasm for promoting and furthering discourse analysis of language to, and by, "ailing" people reinforces my faith in the subject all the time. The faculty members in the English department at the University of Alabama—especially Salli Davis and Catherine Davies—have been most supportive. I am also grateful to the Research Grants Committee at UA for awarding me grant money to do some follow-up research one summer. Elsevier, Guilford Publications, and Cambridge University Press kindly gave me permission to reprint some of my research.

I cannot end this without mentioning the patients and their families who so obligingly found time for me, especially Tina, her husband, and Ellie. Nor can I end without mentioning people whose lives are completely integrated with my own. My parents in India, my uncle and aunt in Los Angeles, my brother in Washington, and my parents-in-law in Georgia all give me that extra hand whenever I slip. Dwight Atkinson—colleague and friend—always holds the other half of all my linguistic ideas; Joe Abbott, my spouse and better half, reminds me always to enjoy the process, and Aasha, my infant daughter, attempts constantly between her naps and feedings to transform me from a grasshopper-researcher into one with slightly more focus. To all these people I am indebted.

1

Introduction

> A new definition of interviewing is proposed and developed in the following chapters that ... centers on a view of the interview as a discourse between speakers and on the ways that the meanings of questions and responses are contextually grounded and jointly constructed by interviewer and respondent ... the aim being to recover and strengthen the voice of the lifeworld, that is, individuals' contextual understandings of their problems in their own terms.
>
> —*Elliot Mishler* (1986a)

This book is about remembering and ways in which it is manifested in particular language use. Most of us go through life not pausing to consider how much of our lives depend on our ability to remember our pasts. Remembering, as Casey (1989) pointed out, goes on continually, often on several levels and in several ways at once. Our memories—especially personal ones—are tied integrally to our identities, to who we are and how we perceive and experience things, people, and the world in general. To fully comprehend the extent to which memory pervades our lives is not really possible. Questions about memory take us into the social environment as well as into people's personal lives.

To realize how critical memory and the act of remembering are, one need only consider instances in which people have lost their ability to remember parts of their pasts. Patients suffering from Alzheimer's disease (AD) are one such population: they constitute the heart of this study. Previous studies examining the language of these patients have been largely psycholinguistic in nature, and their primary focus has been on explaining the patients' deteriorating linguistic skills in terms of failing cognitive skills. Only in recent years has attention been devoted to examining some sociolinguistic dimensions of Alzheimer discourse (Hamilton, 1994; Ramanathan, 1995a, 1995b; Ramanathan-Abbott, 1994; Sabat, 1991), and the present study is an effort at contributing to this growing scholarship.

The direct impetus for this project results from observations and ethnographic notes I made while working as a volunteer in senior day-care centers that cared for AD patients. A noticeable feature was that the language of AD patients seemed more coherent in certain circumstances—with certain people, in certain settings, at certain times—than in others. This led me to investigate ways that variations in contexts influenced the language these patients used and whether differences in their language use could be captured and analyzed in systematic ways. A second motivation for the study stems from my realization that previous psycholinguistic research on Alzheimer's discourse focused, to a large extent, on *language breakdown*, with the discourse being understood in isolation from the context that generated it. In contrast, the present study concentrates on patients' *remnant linguistic skills* by underscoring contextual features of AD discourse. I argue that AD discourse needs to be understood in terms of larger contexts (Hamilton, 1994), specifically the interactions and schemas that generates such discourse. Meaning is not only in the patient's talk, but in the entire context in which the talk is embedded. A third and final motivation has to do with the current state of discourse research. Although several discourse-analytic methods are available and have been employed extensively toward studying a wide range of issues, few of these methods have been applied systematically to the study of "abnormal" discourse. My study not only employs some traditional discourse-analytic methods, but also develops some new analytic concepts by which to study both AD discourse as well other kinds of impaired discourse. These motivations might be better understood if they are observed within the larger context of previous psycholinguistic AD research.

ALZHEIMER'S DISEASE: SOME BACKGROUND INFORMATION

Alzheimer's disease is a kind of dementia that Bayles (1984) defined as a "condition of chronic progressive deterioration of intellect, memory, and communicative function" (p. 209). The term *dementia* signifies a set of behavioral abnormalities often associated with old age. In the late 1800s, Emil Kraeplin (1919) distinguished between two kinds of dementia: senile and presenile dementia. The presenile form of the disease was described by Alois Alzheimer (1907), a neuropathologist, who observed a progressive deterioration of intellect, memory, and orientation in a 51-year-old woman. After her death, Alzheimer discovered cerebral atrophy and the presence of senile plaques and neurofibrillary tangles in her brain.

It is estimated that more than 2 million Americans have AD to the point where they require regular care (Ellis, 1996) and that with baby boomers entering their 50s, the likelihood of individuals with severe dementia will increase by 60% (Light & Lebowitz, 1990). A patient can be said to definitively have AD only on the basis of a biopsy or autopsy of the brain. However, because a biopsy is considered risky, the disease is often diagnosed by eliminating other possible causes, including brain tumors, vitamin deficiencies, and infections (Hamilton, 1994). Katzman (1985) and Reisberg (1981) also included genetic factors, chromosomal abnormalities, dormant viruses, and accumulation of environmental toxins as possible causes.

The clinical course of AD is frequently divided into three relatively distinct phases (Schneck, Reisberg, & Ferris 1982). The first (the *forgetfulness* phase) is characterized by subtle decrements in memory functioning (misplacing objects, difficulty in recalling names). This stage is characterized also by behavioral changes such as decreased spontaneity, social withdrawal, and perhaps anxiety generated by a subjective awareness of failing abilities (Swihart & Pirozzolo, 1988). Language disturbances such as verbal perseverations, halting speech, and mild comprehension deficits are also initial symptoms. During the second stage (the *confusional* phase), cognitive deterioration is more obvious. This stage is marked by such features as obvious memory loss, temporal and spatial disorientation, and poor judgment. Personality changes are also more apparent at this stage. The final stage (the *dementia* phase) is characterized by profound disturbances in orientation and memory, severe intellectual decline, and an inability to recognize even significant persons in the patient's life (e.g., spouse, children). This stage soon progresses to a bedridden state, with limb rigidity and incontinence of urine and feces, and finally death (Swihart & Pirozzolo, 1988).

PSYCHOLINGUISTIC RESEARCH ON ALZHEIMER'S DISEASE

Research devoted to the language abilities of AD patients has increased significantly in recent years. Language dysfunction is a universal concomitant of AD and can occur as the initial symptom of this disorder (Bayles, 1984; Kirshner, Webb, Kelly, & Wells, 1984). Difficulty with lexical retrieval has been widely documented, with object-naming and word-finding difficulties emerging as the most apparent (Appell, Keretz, & Fisman 1982; Schwartz, Martin, & Saffran, 1979). Bayles (1982) found deficits in picture-naming tasks, with subjects producing both semantically related words as well as completely unrelated responses. Bayles and Tomoeda (1983) found that semantically unrelated errors increase with the progression of the disease, and Martin and Fedio (1983), who examined verbal fluency (along with naming), found that subjects produced fewer items and proportionately more superordinate items, compared to normals.

Research on the pragmatic difficulties of these patients, however, have been relatively limited. Most studies have focused on the linguistic deficits of AD patients in experiment-type situations. Hamilton (1994) pointed out that when a "spontaneous" speech component has been studied, it, on the whole, has been elicited in a rigid interview setting, in which the course and development of talk is controlled by the interviewer. Thus, although the subjects in Irigaray's (1973) study were "encouraged to talk about the course of their illness, their profession, and their families," (Obler, 1981, p. 378) the interviewer was in charge.[1] Bayles' (1984) examples of speech from patients in the middle stages of dementia illustrate this (Hamilton, 1994).

In Example 1 the examiner engages the patient in talk by having him or her describe a button:

EXAMPLE 1

> *Examiner:* Tell me everything you can about this (a gray button).
> *Patient:* Oh that's a needle. But ... buttonhole scissors. And they go ahead the put buttons or they put, that's how they put buttons on your coat with it. I guess.

In Example 2, however, the examiner tries to get the patient to explain what it means to "describe" and "guarantee":

EXAMPLE 2

> *Examiner:* What does it mean to describe?
> *Patient:* Well, like you're a buttoning your blouse would be an example.
> *Examiner:* What does it mean to guarantee?
> *Patient:* Guarantee you're gonna get it. I guess we're gonna have company or something. That would be a guarantee, wouldn't it?

(Bayles, 1984, p. 229)

---

[1] Although the present study appears to have the interviewer in charge (as in Bayles' study), I made every effort as an interviewer not to be in charge; I attempted at every stage only to sustain the direction of talk and not to manipulate it.

Hamilton (1994) notes that Bayles' (1984) observations that the patients at this stage are "no longer able to generate verbal sequences of meaningfully related ideas" (p. 228) and that "language becomes egocentric" with less "adherence to the conversational maxims that govern normal conversations" (p. 229) may in fact be valid. However, it is also possible that the patient may not wish to respond simply because he or she does not see the need to talk about a button (Hamiltion 1994; Example 1) or explain "describe" and "guarantee" (Example 2).

Other studies examining the discourse abilities of AD patients have found the patients' language to be low in information. Heir (1985) found that demented subjects made fewer relevant observations, more perseverations, and more incomplete sentences. Nicholas, Obler, and Helm-Estabrooks (1985) found more empty phrases and repetitions, whereas Appell et al. (1982) found that spontaneous AD speech displayed more circumlocutions and semantic jargon. As the dementia progresses, speech becomes increasingly empty with indefinite or generic terms (e.g., "this one," "thing") becoming common. Pronouns without clear reference to antecedents have also been noted (Nicholas et al., 1985).

The narrative abilities of demented patients have been studied by Ulatowska et al. (1988), as well as Ripich and Terrell (1988). Ulatowska et al. examined the narratives of mildly and moderately impaired AD patients to "isolate the linguistic levels at which deficits were evident" (p. 111). Their findings regarding the narrative skills of AD patients included perseveration of the narrative superstructure as well as an inability to produce summaries and morals in narrative discourse. Ripich and Terrell found in their study of cohesion in AD narratives that AD patients use significantly more words and conversational turns. The authors attribute the incoherence in AD speech to the patient's growing inability to take the listener's perspective, and to his or her inability to develop a conversation thematically.

Thus, although there appears to be a substantial body of research in psycholinguistics, there does not appear to be any comparable amount of research done in sociolinguistics. In her groundbreaking book, *Conversations With an Alzheimer's Patient* (1994), Hamilton offered a detailed analysis of an AD patient's deteriorating linguistic skills. Hamilton concluded by stressing the importance of providing Alzheimer patients with rich and stimulating environments so that they feel the need to communicate (p. 166). In her tracing of a patient's deteriorating conversational skills, she called attention to the way her own role as interlocutor changes over time as the responsibility of sustaining coherent conversations falls increasingly on her as the interviewer. Likewise, Sabat (1991) offered a study in which he analyzed how certain types of utterances on his part facilitate more talk from the patient; he demonstrated how, by delaying his own conversational turn, he was able to accommodate the patient's discourse, thereby eliciting coherent speech from the patient.

The present study is similar in many ways to Hamilton's and Sabat's in that it too examines how particular interactional features inhibit extensive and meaningful talk from the patient, whereas others facilitate it. Thus, it reinforces the view that a close examination of language as a social product and process can be another fruitful approach to understanding the Alzheimer experience. Unlike the work of Hamilton and Sabat, however, the present project focuses on the life stories or self narratives of AD patients. Part of the reason for focusing on life stories is because this genre affords extended narrative turns (something that conversation does not necessarily do), thus facilitating an examination of the patients' (in)ability to engage in extended as well as meaningful talk. Previous psycholinguistic research has focused primarily on the *resultant narrative* of patients rather than the *interactional processes* or *schemas* involved in generating the narrative. As the following chapters point out, the ability of a patient to produce and sustain a well-formed narrative varies according to the audience and setting. Indeed, as we see, certain audiences particular audience-moves, and specific settings do *not* facilitate narratives (chaps. 4 and 5). Much narrative production, then, lies in the reciprocal nature of speaking and listening between interactants.

The schematic aspects of AD narratives are illustrated with a focus on the frequent and verbatim repetition of segments of AD talk. Documenting this as a common feature of AD discourse (referred to as *perseveration* in the literature), previous psycholinguistic research has viewed this as a feature that contributes to the meaninglessness of AD discourse. However, by conducting a schematic analysis of the life stories of a patient recorded twice in the span of a year and a half, I point out ways in which these repeated segments, by capturing different life events, have gotten bound and frozen in the teller's memories (Hamilton, 1994) and, also, how the patient's remnant linguistic skills are evident in the connections that the teller has established between life events. Such an approach offers an alternate way of examining the so-called incoherent narratives of patients suffering from AD.

A term that I frequently use in relation to making assessments about patients' discourse abilities is *wellformedness*.[2] "A traditional and bulky term,

---

[2]I need to state here that I have deliberately avoided using the term *coherence* in any technical sense in this study. This is partly because *coherence* has become such a debated notion in discourse analysis, with different scholars establishing different criteria for what constitutes it. Because my expansion of this term would only add to the endless debate surrounding it, I thought it appropriate to unearth the previously used, but now not so common concept of *wellformedness*.

it nevertheless captures a strain central to almost all domains in linguistics, from phonology to syntax to discourse analysis. Linguistics has traditionally been concerned with characterizing wellformed versus deviant strings ..." (Stubbs, 1983, p. 107) and with devising grammars or rules that will predict wellformedness in terms of either syntax or phonemes and morphemes. Such an aim applies to the analysis of spoken discourse as well. Given that the present study is primarily concerned with teasing apart discourse features that facilitate or inhibit wellformed talk from the patient, I feel justified in using this term toward analyzing a chunk of talk. As the following chapters illustrate, wellformedness in this study is assessed primarily in terms of how extensive and meaningful the patients' talk and interactions are. Discourse elements that will enable us to make these judgments are *continuity* and *discontinuity elements*, interactional features that I explain in chapters 2 and 3.

THE DATA FOR THE PRESENT STUDY

The life stories of 16 AD patients—10 females and 6 males—gathered across a span of 5 years constitutes the data for this book. The total number of recorded hours was 36. All of the patients were in the mild to moderate stages of the disease at the time of recording. I recorded the patients in the settings where they spent most of their time: The settings for some were their homes, and for others, their day-care centers. Some of the day-care centers were in poor sections of downtown Los Angeles, where care for the patient was minimal and opportunities for meaningful, communicative activities were sparse. Others were located in posher suburban areas outside Los Angeles where care for the patients was relatively superior, and where staff made efforts to involve the patients in meaningful language use. I note these setting differences because they partially constitute as well as describe the larger context within which the discourse of these patients can be understood, especially the discourse of the two case studies presented in chapters 3, 4, and 5. In all cases, patients were recorded only after I had gotten to know them and their caregivers relatively well.

The life history method was adopted for eliciting narratives in both projects. A life history is "any retrospective account by the individual of his life, in whole or in part, in written or oral form, *that has been elicited or prompted by another person*" (Watson & Watson-Franke, 1985, p. 4, italics added). In all cases, narratives were elicited in as natural a way as possible, allowing the respondent control over the pacing and development of content. That is, the narratives of responses AD patients made to question were to continually inform the evolving interaction. In order to avoid an interview-like atmosphere. I would often find myself sharing parts of my life story with them. I did not have a set of preconceived questions to ask the patients and would generally let them decide the flow and turns of evolving interactions. I would typically start an interaction with a relatively open-ended question such as "when you look back on your past, what is it that stands out most?," and let patients' responses guide me from that point on. In most instances, I would do my best to get them to engage in extended narrative turns. Thus, in instances where they would provide brief responses, I would try to encourage narratives.

The two patients whose life stories and social worlds I analyze in considerable detail are Tina and Ellie. Both were in their mid-60s and both were diagnosed to be in the mild to moderate stages of the disease at the time of recording. Toward establishing that a patient's ability to engage in extended and meaningful talk varies across contexts, Tina's talk was recorded across two audiences (her husband and myself) and two settings (at home and at the day-care center). She was first encouraged to narrate about her past to her husband—to whom she had been married for 32 years, then several hours later to me—she has gotten to know me relatively well. Tina's husband and I both had decided to restrict our questions to specific topics: Tina's childhood, parents, marriages, children, and stay abroad. Both recordings were done at home. I then recorded her in the day-care center a week after the recording at her home.

Ellie, in contrast, was recorded over time, once when she was in the mild to moderate stages of the disease, and then once again a year and a half later when her condition had deteriorated significantly. The analysis in chapter 6 points to ways in which she retained fragments of her overall schema despite her significantly deteriorated state. As the analyses show, I adopt a combination of both micro- and macroethnographic methods toward analyzing both cases. My case study on Tina is relatively more microethnographic because I attempt to see if our interactions, including her ability to narrate, vary across audiences and settings. My study of Ellie, though, has more macroethnographic details because I attempt to show how her linguistic breakdown parallels an increasingly nonfacilitative social context.

Both studies inform my theory of recall laid out in chapter 2. The interactional analyses fall within the realm of what Mishler (1984, 1986) terms *inquiry guided research,* and its primary focus is to concentrate on the interactional *process* involved when eliciting talk. In other words, the process becomes the context for subsequent talk. "Findings ... are examined critically by reflecting on and questioning the assumptions and methods guiding that stage's line of analysis and interpretation" (Mishler, 1984, p.

13). The analysis in the present study includes both an examination of narratives, and a critical look at interactional engagements between myself and the patients. Indeed, as the following chapters point out, there are certain moves at certain points in the interactions where I, as audience and researcher, inhibit the patient's ability to engage in extended and meaningful talk. Such an approach—what I call reflexive researching—allows me to turn the critical lens on myself to investigate how *I* as researcher and audience contribute to the relative "incoherence" in patient talk.

"The value of rhetorical self-awareness is in drawing our attention to the constructions through which, as professionals, we have learned partly to read, but which still masks many difficult and misleading assumptions about the purpose and politics of our work" (Myers, 1988, p. 622). Such a mode of analysis, I believe, truly "directs attention to the ways that values are embedded in assumptions about methods and theory" (Mishler, 1984, p. 14).

Schematic analysis, however, is the kind of analysis adopted most often by cognitive anthropologists. It explores how the discourse of narrators points to ways in which information (about oneself or about the world) is cognitively represented in the brain and how such representation informs ways by which people interpret human behavior. Recent research by D'Andrade (1992) and Strauss (1992) shows how schemas are evident in talk as well as the ways in which these schemas serve to structure and order people's views and values. Both kinds of analysis are appropriate to this study in that they allow us to locate and understand narrative wellformedness in terms of larger frameworks; both kinds of analysis enable us to see that all resultant talk needs to be understood in terms of larger contexts within which it is embedded.

OVERVIEW OF THE CHAPTERS

Chapter 2 lays out the theoretical framework for this study: the complex equation between recall, reminding and self-narratives; and the criteria for gauging narrative and interactional wellformedness. Focusing primarily on the data, chapter 3 is devoted to examining wellformedness in terms of both patient and audience talk. Wellformedness in patient talk is assessed chiefly in terms of whether the narratives lend themselves to stanza parsing, and interactional wellformedness in terms of both *kinds* and *positioning* of audience turns and whether they succeed in engaging the patient in recall. The chapter begins with a general discussion of these features in Tina's life stories before moving on to address features evident in the larger data pool.

Chapter 4 examines narrative and interactional illformedness. Like chapter 3, it begins with an in-depth analysis of Tina's talk, focusing on her inability to narrate and the nature of some of my turns that inhibit her recalling process. I then address how the relative positioning of my turns across the data pool hinders AD patients from engaging in narrative turns. Chapter 5 is also devoted to examining Tina's talk, but this time across audiences: her husband Nick and myself. The chapter calls attention to the fact that the illformed nature of Tina's talk is a result partly from Nick's extensive repair utterances that contribute to rendering their interaction discontinuous. The analysis also points out how Nick seems to engage Tina in recognition, an activity, that like his repair utterances, is not conducive to narrative development.

Chapter 6 explores some discourse implications of unitized chunks of talk in AD discourse that get repeated over and over again. Although repetition generally has been seen to contribute to "incoherence" in AD talk, this chapter points out how these repeated segments make sense when understood as part of a larger schema. By doing a schematic analysis of Ellie's life stories, I show how the bound and unbound events get linked to each other and to her overall schema. By offering ethnographic details of her life and social world, I attempt to draw parallels between her exacerbating condition and her nonfacilitative environment. Finally, chapter 7 discusses some implications of this study. The implications for psycholinguistic research include the importance of using natural data elicited in relatively unstructured situations (Hamilton, 1994) and the ways in which the analyses inform the notion of "learned helplessness" (Lubinski, 1991). The chapter also addresses the importance of having AD patients recall their pasts as well as some ways of training caregivers to hear their patients' cues.

As a final word, because the study has implications for a variety of disciplines—including discourse analysis, communication, and gerontology—I have tried to keep my style as jargon-free as possible. As its audience, this book seeks all who are interested in Alzheimer discourse and the complex equation between memory, language use, and contextual features. It offers at its center an examination of some communicative strategies that do and do not work with Alzheimer patients, people whose memories are increasingly fragile and slipping away.

Transcript notations are as follows:

> [...] (pauses): indicated by dots in square brackets with the number of dots corresponding to the number of seconds.
> . (period): marking closure with a falling intonation
> , (comma splice): marking a brief fall in voice indicating that more information is to follow.
> CAPITAL letters: emphasis.

2

Theoretical Framework

> At certain moments in life, prompted by the excitement of some major event, we look ahead in time and think quite simply, "I shall remember this forever." And this awareness in itself seems to change the present experience, to enhance it like some object being lit suddenly from a new side. These are among the very few times that we have direct and honest contact with our future selves. Otherwise we are largely, and in a sense unnecessarily, exiled from our own future.
>
> —*Robert Grudin* (1982)

The quote from Grudin's *The Time and Art of Living* has several interesting implications regarding how we "invent" ourselves (Bruner & Weisser, 1991) through the life stories we tell. The idea of "major events" calls to mind Linton's (1987) idea of "significant memories," (1982), memories that critically inform the kind of story(ies) we tell about ourselves. It also makes us aware of the temporal dimensions, the simultaneously present and past nature, if you will, of our life stories: Although they are about our pasts, they are, at the moment of telling, rooted in the present. Implied also is the genre of (re)telling: It is, in most cases, a narrative (Tonkin, 1992).

All of these implications are central to the discussion in this chapter. The life story as a form revolves around notions of identity and self (Bruner & Weisser, 1991); the question, "Who am I?" is at the heart of the life story genre although it is not necessarily a question overtly acknowledged by tellers. That is, tellers do not necessarily tell their life stories in response to "Who are you?" or proceed with "I am going to tell you who I am" (although these prompts cannot be ruled out). They are more likely to tell them in more naturalistic occasions as when a group of people are exchanging stories about certain times in their lives.

Regardless, at least for the moment, of how the life story emerges, the question "Who am I?" has particular implications for the elderly. As Sherman (1991) put it, the elderly are likely to frame this question as "Who have

I been all this time?" When we consider that the aging process brings with it withdrawal from the work world and increased losses of relatives, friends, and loved ones as well as actual decrease in physical energy—all of which have been tied to one's sense of self—then "the impulse to remember and evoke the memories and images of these lost objects is understandable (Sherman, 1991, p. 7). For the elderly person suffering from AD,[1] the question of "Who am I?" becomes increasingly difficult in that memory and language skills so crucial to inventing a self are progressively deteriorating.

In general, reminiscence or reconstructing one's past has been understood to play a valuable role in the lives of the elderly (Sherman, 1991). The act of narrating one's past or reconstructing one's autobiography can be seen to serve two functions. First, it is an act of clarifying and sorting out events and experiences, which at the moment of telling are, on the whole, a disorganized mass of thoughts.[2] It is also an act of making sense of one's past in the realm of actual experience. Second, it is an act of putting oneself together, an act of constructing a picture of oneself or as Radley (1990) stated, an act of establishing one's biographical identity. Both of these acts—self construction and making sense—are related: The act of making sense of one's past is actually the act of constructing oneself. Polkinghorne's view (1988) that "we achieve our personal identities and self-concept through narrative configuration and make our existence into a whole by understanding it as an expression of a single unfolding and developing story" (p. 150) can be viewed as an effective summing up of both these functions of narrating. Working through troublesome and painful memories, especially those that become obsessive and take on lives of their own, is particularly important for the elderly if they want to retain and present a past or self that has as few disjunctions as possible (Coupland et al., 1991).

Self-narrative or autobiographical reconstruction crucially depends on memory, because our ability to reconstruct our pasts depends on our ability to remember past experiences. However, this does not mean that we are able to recall every single incident and detail accurately and vividly, or even that we are able to recall the exact chronological sequence of events.[3] In

---

[1] All of the patients who participated in the study were at least 65 years of age or older.

[2] This is not to say that all our memories are disorganized before we construct them in narrative form. All of us have, to varying degrees, memories that have been well rehearsed, memories that have been previously made sense of and that tend to be recounted in the same way each time they are recalled.

[3] Bartlett (1932) believed that remembering, like recognition, depends on perception. Perception, according to him, is a "sensory function" and has a "psychological orientation and attitude" (p. 193). Remembering has these features, but it is distinct inasmuch as "material remembered usually has to be set in relation with other material, and in most complete cases has to be dated, placed, and given some kind of personal mark" (p. 195). The ability and accuracy with which we recall depends on the intensity with which we have perceived and absorbed that event.

fact, none of us, when we are asked to narrate spontaneously our life stories for the first time, are aware of the exact sequence of events as they occurred in our lives.[4] That is, we do not have the order mapped out in our heads before we begin narrating. Rather, the act of narrating provides the order and the sequence. The casting of events in a linear narrative form, then, is crucial to the (re)construction of our pasts.

There are some memories that are more significant than others. The significant memory has what Linde (1987) called *extended reportability*. That is, this memory is likely to be recalled every time the life story is told.[5] Although the teller may have made sense of the event in the past (in previous recountings of it), he or she may occasionally make fresh sense of it in the light of newer, more recent experiences. (This, however, does not apply to well-rehearsed memories whose interpretations, on the whole, tend to remain unchanged.) The sense the teller may have made of it previously would have been governed by a whole range of social factors (time, place, occasion, audience) most of which will not be the same the next time the event is recalled.

The idea that our life stories change depending on context raises questions regarding how we (especially researchers) assess accuracy in life stories. One way to test verisimilitude would be to compare the teller's initial representation of a story with subsequent representations but, as Ross and Buehler (1994) pointed out, the problem with this method of verification is that the two representations could reflect very different but equally compelling depictions of reality. Gaining consensus over different interpretations of life events could be another way of testing for accuracy, but agreement does not necessarily mean truth. "The history of science reveals that consensually accepted truths of today are often overturned tomorrow" (Ross & Buehler, 1994, p. 68). Disagreement about interpretations, however, could serve a useful function in that it would serve to make one skeptical of the different stories. But once again, gaining a skeptical orientation does not necessarily enable one to arrive at the truth. How then do discourse analysts judge the accuracy of their own and others' memories?

Bruner's ideas (1986) on narrative thought are relevant here. Bruner maintained that a well-constructed narrative thought is (a) vivid and

---

[4]Neisser (1982) has an article on the "nested structure" of autobiographical memory. According to him smaller "molecular" events are nested in larger "molar" ones; recall is almost always a construction of "molar" events.

[5]Linton (1982) characterized two features of those events that endure in memory: (a) "The event must be salient and be perceived as strongly emotional at the time it occurs," and (b) "the event may be seen as a turning point, the beginning of a sequence or as instrumental in other later activities" (p. 89).

detailed rather than sketchy; (b) coherent in that the events are sequenced and connected in an intuitively plausible manner; and (c) characterologically consistent, with characters' actions seeming to stem from their personalities, intentions, and motives. A gripping story can be true even though the characters and events are fictional. These characteristics of narrative thought can be seen to apply to the analysis of life stories: Life stories and personal memories can be assessed as true if they are vivid, detailed, and consistent, and especially, given the criteria for the present study, if they are extensive and meaningful (and thus wellformed).

We turn now to discussing some possible ways that Meacham (1994) laid out regarding how to conceive of the remembering process. The first approach stresses factual accuracy as crucial to the remembering process, in which the teller's ability to remember and account for events exactly as they happened is of central importance. Important in this view is the degree to which a particular memory corresponds with the event in the past (p. 39). Remembering, in this approach, is conceived of as emerging and generating from the mind of the individual, with the individual in complete control over his or her memories. A problem with this approach to remembering is that if the teller is not able to remember, then he or she is considered deficient or lacking in some way.

The second approach to the remembering process is "discovering the meaning of memories" (p. 40), wherein what is stressed is whether the individual can arrive a plausible understanding regarding the meanings of memories. Factual recall or the ability of the teller to recall facts in a verbatim manner, then, is relatively deemphasized in this approach. However, as Meacham warned, this approach can lead to viewing the teller as distorting memories or at least discovering meanings in memories to suit the needs of the immediate context.

Finally, the third approach to remembering attempts to construct the meaning of memories. Here remembering is seen to have the power "to bring into existence specific remembered details that appear to serve as support for the meaning"(p. 43). Such an approach to life stories, especially those of AD patients, allows the discourse analyst/researcher to begin articulating life themes—or overall schemas as I refer to them—that the patient is unable to do for him or herself. As the analysis in chapter 6 points out, Ellie's speech indicates connections to her overall schemas despite her deteriorated condition.

The approach to remembering adopted in this volume is partially a combination of the last two processes of remembering. I take the view that remembering is simultaneously a process of both discovering and constructing memories and their meaning(s) by teller and researcher, a process that occurs in contexts of ongoing interactions. The patients' inability to engage in recall or to construct a wellformed story of their pasts, then, is partially an interactional one: The contributions of the audience may either facilitate or impede the patients' recalling process. The process is also significantly influenced by the tellers' overall schemas that indicate how they have made sense of their pasts. Such an approach shifts attention away from the view that memories are located in the individual's head to a view of remembering that is co-constructed and social. Indeed, if we did not acknowledge the social aspects of our remembering processes, "we would be in continual conflict with each other as we held fast to our convictions that our own, individual memories were the only faithful copies of past events" (Meacham, 1994, p. 45).

RECALL, REMINDING, AND RECOGNITION

I would like now to address the notions of *recall, reminding,* and *recognition* and the ways in which I use these (everyday) terms for the remainder of the book. *Recall,* as far as this volume is concerned, is the tellers' ability to render (orally) their past in narrative form. As mentioned earlier, one of my aims in this volume is to gauge both the extent to which patients' are able to engage in (self) narrative turns and the influence that different audiences and settings have on this ability. This meant that as researcher and audience I was—in several interactions—trying to provide turns, prompts, and utterances that would engage the Alzheimer's disease (AD) patients in recall (and narrative turns). As some of the analysis points out, I was not always successful. In chapters 3 and 4, I show how the relative positioning of some of my utterances in the ongoing interactions seem to influence the patients' (in)ability to recall. Likewise the case study on Tina (chaps. 3, 4, and 5) points out how her husband's turns inhibit her narrative process. Given the general layout of the present study then, recall, as a discourse activity, appears to have the following characteristics:

1. It takes a narrative form; the tellers are generally able to engage in extended and meaningful turns about past events.
2. Tellers generally bear the onus of retrieving and selecting the memories they wish to talk about.
3. Tellers are able to integrate the turns of the audiences' into their ongoing stories. In other words, audience turns do not derail the teller's ongoing turn (or thought processes); instead, they serve a facilitative function.

Reminding, though, is quite different. If recall has partially to do with retrieving of and deciding on previously stored information, then reminding has to do with *establishing relatedness between units of stored information*. Whereas recall also involves establishing relatedness, it is, as we shall see, a relatively more integrated activity than reminding. We are reminded of one person by another, of one occasion by another, or of one object by another. But more importantly and particularly relevant to the present study is that reminding as an activity occurs across situations with one life event reminding tellers of others and where tellers do not go into detail about connected life events (whereas in recall, as we just noted, tellers do go into detail about specific memories). Schank (1980) distinguished between the following classes of reminding:

1. Physical objects can remind you of other physical objects.
2. Physical objects can remind you of events.
3. Events can remind you of physical objects.
4. Events can remind you of events in the same domain.
5. Events can remind you of events in different domains. (p. 20)

The last two classes in this list most directly inform the current discussion on life events. Why one life event reminds us of another is of primary importance because it sheds light, not only on what units of information have been stored together, but more pertinently on the tellers' sensemaking process when they are engaged in reconstructing their pasts. Given the assumption that making sense of a life event means "finding an appropriate place for a representation of that event in memory" (Schank, 1980, p. 20), then reminding would indicate that a particular life event has been triggered in the process of remembering. For this to happen, we either have to be looking to be reminded (of a particular life event), which signals a degree of conscious effort on the part of the teller, or we have to run into it accidently, which does not necessarily imply conscious effort on the teller's part.

Given the data for the study, it would appear that both these explanations help us understand why AD patients are sometimes able to integrate the reminded event into their ongoing story and why at other times they seem stymied. As we shall presently see, patients sometimes need to be prompted into recalling with audience turns that encourage them to make connections between life events, whereas at other times they are able to manage on their own. In both cases, audiences seem to have an integral role to play. As a discourse activity then, reminding can be characterized as an activity in which (a) tellers are able to establish relatedness between life events but are unable to integrate the reminded event into their ongoing story (generally once they begin integrating the reminded life event into their story, the discourse activity the discourse activity becomes recall) and (b) audience turns impede patients from engaging in recall/narrative turns.

We turn now to discuss *recognition* as another relevant memory process. It might be helpful if I begin by pointing out how recognition differs from recall, at least in experimental psychological research. As Brown (1976) states, a recall test is one in which "the subject has to generate the target or targets meeting the definition of the target in the recall instruction" (p. 1). This target may or may not be a part of a well-defined set. If the target is a word, the testee may have to speak or write it; if it is a picture or an idea, he or she is often asked to describe or draw it. The segment cited from Bayles (1984) in chapter 1 wherein she had an AD describe a gray button is an example of such a recall test.

A recognition test, however, is one in which the testee response consists of accepting or rejecting a given choice. In some recognition tests, the testee is also required to rate the item, connect it to other choices present, or in a multiple choice test, choose the most plausible item (Brown, 1976). A factor likely to influence recognition is the memorability of the presented item, which, as Gee (1992) pointed out, depends on the way in which it is "tagged" to the other events in the testee's (teller's) mind. (This point regarding how information gets tagged and stored becomes clearer in the section on schemas). The tester provides the testee with a "code" that facilitates recognition. In other words, the code acts as a stimulus for the retrieval of a set of tagged items from the testee's memory. In the light of the present discussion, certain kinds of audience turns and prompts serve as codes that trigger recognition of a life event and ultimately recall.

Another important distinction between recognition and recall has to do with the contextual element embedded in each. As Tulving (1976) pointed out, recall involves much more of the *contextual* element than recognition does. Hollingworth (1913) captured this distinguishing element:

> Recall is that aspect of memory process in which a *setting*, a background or association cluster is present in clear consciousness, but the desired *focal element* is missing.... In recognition the focal element is present in the form of sensation, image or feeling and the question is not whether this element will recall a more or less definite setting or background ... (1913, pp. 532–533).

Hollingworth does not just describe the differences between recall and recognition as methods of measuring retention. He also points to differences in the underlying process. Theorists like Norman (1968) also believe that the contextual element is what distinguishes recall from recognition. Both processes involve an association between item and context, but whereas the task in recognition is to proceed from the item to the context, the task in recall is the reverse, to generate the item given its context (Norman, 1968; Tulving, 1976).

Formalizing the differences between recognition and recall, Kintsch (1970) said that recall involves the stages of *retrieval* and *decision*, whereas recognition involves only the latter. He noted that in recognition "the item is sensorily present and it is a simple matter to retrieve its corresponding representation in memory." In recall, the items/stimuli are not present, but they must be retrieved from memory, and "retrieval involves getting from one memory trace to the next" (Kintsch, 1970, p. 337). Other versions of this two-stage process have been proposed by Anderson and Bower (1972, 1974). In terms of the interactions studied for the present project, then, recognition can be characterized as a discourse activity in which (a) the audience holds up a particular life event (target item) to the teller, and (b) audience turns are such that the teller is not able to engage in a narrative turn, with (b), in most cases, resulting from (a).

As for distinguishing between recognition and reminding, in order for the patient to be engaged in recognition, the audience must know of (significant) life events in the teller's pasts so as to hold them up to the teller; that is, the audience and teller must have fairly extensive shared knowledge. Indeed, the analyses of some interactions between Tina and N (chap. 5) and between Ellie and me (chap. 7) point to ways in which N and I, as audiences, unconsciously hold up target events for the patients to recognize. Because we are aware of some details about their pasts, we draw on that knowledge to trigger recall from them, but as the analyses point out, we are not successful because our prompts end up engaging them in recognition. This is not the case, however, when the patient is engaged in reminding and where the audience need not have any shared knowledge with the teller at all. In such cases, the audience makes turns that prompt the patient into self-reminding (detailed in chap. 3) or turns that trigger connected life events that sometimes do and sometimes do not get integrated into the teller's ongoing stories.

Reminding ———————————————————————— Recall
Recognition

FIG. 2.1. Recall, reminding, and recognition as discourse activities on a narrative continuum.

In summary, we could conceive of the three activities—reminding, recognition, and recall—as occupying different points on a narrative continuum (see Fig. 2.1).

Given that one of my aims in this study was to engage patients in extended and meaningful speech, I was, in effect, constantly attempting to pull the interaction from reminding and recognition to recall. I do need to note here that these activities are by no means mutually exclusive: Much of reminding and recognition is entailed in recall, and much of recall is a result of reminding and recognition. My presenting them as seemingly dichotomous activities is done in an effort to clarify audience roles, showing how particular audience turns seem to engage patients in different activities.

GAUGING NARRATIVE AND INTERACTIVE WELLFORMEDNESS

One of the issues lurking beneath the discussion thus far is how one judges whether patients are engaged in recall and ways of assessing wellformedness of talk. One way of assessing *narrative wellformedness* is by determining whether the patient's talk lends itself to stanza segmentation (Gee, 1991). Of course, whether stanza segmentation is possible depends, to a large extent, on whether the interaction facilitates extended and meaningful talk from the patient. Toward gauging interactive wellformedness, I examine whether the interaction evidences continuity and discontinuity elements, features that partially serve both to keep the interaction on track and to encourage more talk from the patient (thus facilitating chances of recall).

Recall and Narrative Wellformedness: Stanzas

A stanza can best be thought of as a cohesive device that is particularly suitable for assessing extended pieces of talk such as narratives. Claiming that stanzas are universal, Gee (1990) believed that they are "the products of the mental mechanism by which humans produce speech" (p. 117), and that "these structures reflect units of human narrative/discourse competence" (p. 125). He defined the stanza as a set of "lines" (clauses or simple sentences), usually about a single minimal topic, organized rhythmically and syntactically to form a discourse unit, thus serving as a cohesive function. Each stanza can be seen to indicate a shift in action, character, participants, or time such that when character, place, time, event, or the function of a piece of information changes (whether in an argument, report, exposition, or description), the stanza must change (Gee, 1990, p. 106).

In many ways, a stanza structure can be seen as a transcribing technique that tries to capture both the prosody of the speaker's talk and the text's thematic structure. Here is the way it works on the following excerpt from Labov and Waletzsky (1966). The number to the right marks the number of each stanza:

I *talked a man out of*—Old Doc Simon, I *talked him out of* pulling the trigger.	1
In the business I was associated at that time the Doc was an old man. He had killed one man or had done time.	2
But he had a young wife, and those days I dressed *well*. And seemingly she was trying to make me.	3
I never noticed it, fact is, I didn't like her very *well*. Because she—she was a nice looking girl until you saw her *feet*, she had *big feet*, Jesus God, she had *big feet*! (p. 294)	4

Because this excerpt (like the data for this study) is a written version of an oral text, we have little sense of the *prosody* of the teller's speech, the way in which the speaker's voice rose and fell in pitch, the way in which he lengthened and shortened his syllables, the way in which he speeded up and slowed down his rate of speech, and the places where he hesitated and paused. These features not only convey the speaker's attitudes, views, motives, and emotions, they also constitute the overall rhythm of the piece of talk. One way in which these oral features can be partially captured in a written text is by devising or using written markings that attempt to "capture what the voice is doing" (Gee, 1991, p. 106).

Lines and stanzas attempt to do this. Let us briefly consider the ways in which they can be identified. In the preceding excerpt, the period at the end of a line signifies a fall in the pitch of the voice, a *closure* (considered by the speaker to be complete or finished). Gee referred to such a pitch movement as a *closure contour*. A comma at the end of a line, however, stands for a slight rise or fall in pitch. This signals, not the closure of information, but that more information is to follow. Gee refers to this as a *continuation contour*. A set of topically related lines/ideas constitutes a stanza, which, as mentioned earlier, can be identified around a shift in focus, character, perspective, and action.

The stanza structure also permits us to see the continuity between the ideas in the text. The first stanza in the preceding excerpt lays out briefly what the narrative is about ("I talked ... Old Doc Simon ... out of pulling the trigger"). The second stanza elaborates on this not only by using more detail, but also by providing a concrete example ("He had killed one man or had done time"). In the third stanza, we see a shift in perspective: The narrator suddenly moves from talking about Old Doc to talking about Old Doc's wife, who was making passes at him ("And seemingly she was trying to make me"). The fourth stanza, while elaborating on the ideas introduced in the third stanza, also indicates a shift in perspective in which the narrator defends why he was not attracted to her ("she had *big feet*, Jesus God/she had *big feet!*").

This kind of parsing is effective in judging whether and to what degree the AD patients studied here are able to engage in recall. Because each stanza is made up of topically related sets of lines, it allows us to break down the overall narrative structure in small increments. This "unpackaging" of the structure enables us to see the continuity/connectedness between the ideas, thereby facilitating a view of the discourse organization of the text. It also permits us to glean the meaning in the narrative. Because each stanza is topically/thematically related to other stanzas, unpackaging enables us to see how the different stanzas together contribute to the overall thematic unity, and by extension, to the wellformedness of the text.

Recall and Interactive Wellformedness: Continuity Elements

Because narrative production is an interactive phenomenon in that a narrative in most cases is coproduced, conversation-analytic tools used to study the sequential, continuous nature of conversations have been applied to studying interactions with extended (story) turns as well (Bauman, 1986; Mandelbaum, 1989; Mishler, 1984). A primary characteristic of Western conversation is its ongoing nature, with participants sequencing their turns. Talk is designed to reflect back on prior turns and project ahead to future ones, and we interpret talk as if it were tied in some way to prior and future turns. Central to conversation-analytic research is the notion of all utterances being understood "by reference to their placement and participation within sequences of actions" (Heritage, 1984, p. 5): Sequences and turns within sequences are the primary units of analysis. Every turn in an ongoing conversation projects a relevant next action or range of actions to be accomplished by the next participant in his or her next turn, an event generically referred to as *sequential implicativeness*. One way in which this is often accomplished is through the production of the first pair part of an *adjacency pair* (sequences such as question–answer, greeting–greeting). However, once we have recognized that some current or first action projects some appropriate second, "it becomes relevant to examine the various ways in which a second speaker may accomplish such a second, or analyzably withhold its accomplishment, or avoid its accomplishment by undertaking some other activity" (Heritage, 1984, p. 6). The first part of a sequence then projects onto the next participant "a pressure" to "tie-up" his or her utterance to the previous one (largely in terms of making a topically related utterance). It is this pressure to link utterances to prior turns that generates *continuity* in the ongoing talk. The following fragment from Heritage (1984) cited in Nofsinger (1991) illustrates this:

> Don: I like that blue one very much
> Sam: And I'll bet your wife would like it
> Don: If I had the money I'd get one for her
> Sam: And one for your mother I'll bet (Heritage, 1984, transcript notation)

There is continuity in Sam's utterances in that they are topically related to Don's utterances. Sam's utterance "I'll bet your wife would like it" relates directly back to Don's utterance about the blue dress, while also projecting Don's next turn ("If I had the money I'd get one for her"), which, in turn, projects Sam's next turn ("And one for your mother I'll bet").

Turn exchanges in narrative interactions operate a little differently from the way they do in conversations. "Stories, as told in conversation, are produced through routine conversational processes and integrated with other conversational structures" (Nofsinger, 1991, p. 155). Very much a part of everyday talk, they are *locally occasioned* by one or more conversational turns (Jefferson, 1978). An utterance by one interlocutor may trigger a narrative, and the teller, in conjunction with the audience, will construct the story. Thus, by turn exchanges (Sacks, 1974) between teller and listener, the story takes shape. However, in conversations with embedded stories, the teller takes more extended turns than in conversations without stories (e.g., as in exchanging pleasantries). "Despite recipient's participation being often minimal in *quantitative* terms, conversational analysts' accounts show how the turns that recipients take are instrumental in the storytelling coming to the floor" (Mandelbaum, 1989, p. 116).

The telling of most stories is prefaced with an interaction, an exchange of speaker turns, as when the teller signals the recipient about an imminent story: "Did you hear what happened?" "No, tell me" (followed by the narrative), or when one interactant specifically prompts another interactant into telling a story: "Tell me about a memorable experience"; "Okay, I'll tell you about something that happened in my childhood" (followed by a narrative). This illustrates one way in which narrating is interactional. The recipient's utterances can have important consequences, not just on the *way* a story is told, but on *what* is told as well. Had the recipient in the preceding (second) instance changed his or her mind and said, "No, don't tell me something that happened in your childhood; tell me about a *recent* memorable experience," the teller's story would likely have been very different from the one he or she may have chosen in response to the previous prompt. The recipient's prompt is crucial, then, in generating particular kinds of narratives.

Once the teller has begun the narrative, the recipient has to play a role toward sustaining the continuity of the narrative, and as Mandelbaum (1989) pointed out, this is also interactive. Although the onus of storytelling falls on the teller, there are places in the exchange where the recipient takes turns. These recipient turns, when plotted on a continuum, could range from passive participation, in which the recipient does not "interfere" with the story (implicit in the recipient's silence is the "go-ahead" signal to the teller to keep talking) to turns that affirm the teller's talk (continuers such as "uh huh," "mm hmm," "oh ya?") to turns that could extend talk (like collaborative turns) to utterances that could completely derail the teller's current turn (by initiating a new topic, for instance), or at least could threaten it by extended pauses or excessive repair turns (as the present study points out). In some cases the particular positioning of audience turns in ongoing interactions also contributes to facilitating narratives or inhibiting them. Figure 2.2 is a visual representation of this.

I refer to these audience turns as continuity and discontinuity elements (depending on the nature and function of the recipient turn). Those that

Continuity devices   Discontinuity devices

| Silence | sustainers | collaboratives | pauses | repair |

FIG. 2.2. Relative positioning of audience turns.

serve to maintain and encourage continuity both in the emerging narrative and in the interaction are continuity elements, whereas those that impede the narrator's extended turn, thereby rendering the narrative and interaction discontinuous, are discontinuity elements. We turn now to reviewing some continuity elements that, although traditionally applied in conversation-analytic research, can be effectively applied to Alzheimer interactions. Many of these are adapted from Nofsinger (1991), who addressed some of these elements in terms of alignment in conversations. (Discontinuity elements are addressed in the following chapters.)

Assessments

One way by which recipients establish continuity in interactions is by *assessing* the previous turn. When the previous turn has conveyed information, the next turn is often in the form of an evaluative statement that conveys whether the previous turn has communicated good or bad news. The following segment demonstrates what I mean:

C:	How's yer *foot*.	1
A:	Oh it's healing beautifully:	2
C:	Goo::d	3

(Heritage, 1985, cited in Nofsinger, 1991, p. 115)

C's response in Line 3 demonstrates her tying up her utterance to A's prior turn: She is responding to A's utterance as if it conveyed good news, thus continuing the interaction. However, because we do not know A's counterresponse to C, we are in no position to tell whether C's "Goo::d" was the appropriate response. As Nofsinger (1991) pointed out, it is quite possible that A does not want her foot to heal "beautifully." If we knew what A's next utterance was, we would be better able to tell if her utterance sustained the continuity that C's assessment initiated.

Newsmarkers

Recipients also respond to new information, announcements, and reports in ways that underscore informational value. Conversational elements that do this are newsmarks, words or expressions that view the previous turn as newsworthy for the recipient (Heritage, 1984). They include expressions such as "really?," my goodness," and partial repeats of prior turns (e.g., "she did?"). Produced sometimes to express surprise, they serve to encourage the previous speaker to keep talking about the (newsworthy) topic and in this sense serve to continue the interaction. In the following segment a "normal" elderly woman talks to me about a restaurant she recently had visited:

A:	It was pretty bad	1
I:	Oh really? Bad huhh?	2
A:	Yea:: I though:t so	3
I:	What'd you ha::ve?	4

My utterances on Line 2 are both newsmarks and partial repeats that further talk by encouraging A to continue her thoughts about the restaurant.

Another kind of newsmark is the "oh receipt" also studied by Heritage (1984). Occasionally used alone and sometimes used with other newsmarks, "oh", as Heritage proposes functions as a change-of-state token, displaying that the user has changed from being an uninformed interactant to being an informed one. In this way "oh" not only extends interaction but confirms that both speaker and recipient knowledge is now changed with the (speaker's) new information. The following segment illustrates this point:

J:	Hello ther I rang y'earlier but chu wur ou:t	1
K:	*Oh*: I musta been at *Dez'z mu:m's*	2
J:	==Oh::.	3
	(Nofsinger, 1991, p. 117)	

In Line 1, we see J informing K of an earlier phone call (Line 1); the assumption of K's ignorance of this matter is articulated in "but chu wur out." In Line 3, K combines an "Oh" receipt with an account of why she was not able to take J's call. The "oh" here (Line 2) indicates that K had been unaware of J's call, but is now informed. We see a similar change-of-information state in J when he responds with "oh": Now he is the one who undergoes a change-of-information state, because he is now informed about why K did not answer his call. Continuation is achieved in the way that both participants adjust to their newly informed states.

Sustainers

Similar to newsmarks and "oh" receipts are *sustainers* such as like "mm hmm" or "uh huh" and "yah" that demonstrate that the listener is listening and, in some cases, understanding what the speaker is saying. According to Schegloff (1982), speakers who use these elements in interactions avoid taking a full turn; they display their understanding in recognizing that the other speaker is building an extended turn and should continue with the next unit of it. We see this in the following modified segment:

```
H:    One time I remember, .hh's girl wrote              1
      and her,.hh she wz like (.) fifteen er             2
      six teen and her mother doesn't let'er wear        3
      [       ]
N:    Uh hu:h,                                           4
H:    .hh nail polish ...                                5
(Nofsinger, 1991, p. 119)
```

Although N's sustainer in Line 4 inhibits H from completing her full turn, it allows N to demonstrate her recognition that H is in the middle of her story as well as her cooperation in allowing H to continue. In doing so, N facilitates H's extended turn, thereby furthering their interaction.

Formulations

Formulations are continuity devices by which a participant will summarize or give a gist of what some other participant said (Nofsinger, 1991), with some responses being immediate and others delayed. In many ways these devices perform a function similar to "so-summary statements" (Ferrara, 1994) in therapeutic discourse in that they indicate what the recipient has comprehended from the speaker's previous turn. Citing Heritage (1985) Nofsinger explained that formulations need not necessarily be comprehensive or neutral summaries of prior talk. In some cases, the recipient may choose to focus only on certain parts of the teller's turn. In the following segment (cited in Nofsinger, 1991), a woman who has won a dieting award (Slimmer of the Year) is being interviewed:

```
S:   ... .I never ever felt my age or looked my age,=I was      1
     always (.) older,=people always took me for older..hhhh    2
     And when I was at college I think I looked a ma:tronly     3
     fifty.. hh And (.) I was completely alone one weekend and I 4
     got to this stage where I almost jumped in the river(hh).=I 5
     just felt life wasn't worth it anymo:re,                   6
     =it hadn't anything to offer (.).hhhand if this was living I 7
     had had enough                                             8
I:   You really were prepared to commit suicide because you     9
     were a big fatty                                          10
S:   Yes, cuz I-I(.) just didn't see anything in life that I   11
     had to look forward to ...                                12
(Heritage, 1985, p. 101)
```

The interviewer's formulations in Lines 9 and 10 selectively focus on some of S's utterance. We see that she captures the main point of S's turn and says it in her own words: "You really were prepared to commit suicide because you were a big *fatty*." In doing so, the recipient demonstrates her understanding of what is important in the speaker's prior turn; by highlighting or confirming (or disconfirming as the case may be) an aspect of the speaker's prior turn(s), the recipient continues the interaction.

Collaborations

A *collaborated completion* is a continuity device whereby a recipient anticipates the completion of the prior speaker's turn and completes the utterance for the speaker. The following is an example from one of my interactions with a "normal" elderly:

S: If you didn't follow her rules
V: it meant you didn't belong
(R at home, June, 1992)

Lerner (1989) maintains that the organization or the syntax of certain utterances allows the listener(s) to anticipate how the utterance will be completed. The recipient then guesses the direction the turn will take and completes the first speaker's utterance. In the preceding instance, my preemptive completion of S's turn becomes a way by which I indicate to I that I understand her prior turn; it also allows me to communicate my interest in continuing the interaction.

In summary, then, various types of continuity devices are evident in all sequential talk (depending on how speakers have interpreted prior talk). Newsmarks and "Oh" receipts display the newsworthy value of prior talk, whereas assessments show whether recipients have interpreted prior talk to be good or bad. Formulations demonstrate what the recipient thinks is worth highlighting (in the prior turn) in his or her summary, whereas collaborative completions show how recipients anticipate the end of an utterance. Sustainers likewise indicate the recipient's recognition of the prior speaker's extended turn. Thus, through these elements participants continually demonstrate involvement in the ongoing interaction, thereby furthering talk. As we see presently, these elements contribute to the patients' abilities to engage in recall.

SUMMING UP

Recall, narratives, stanzas, interactions, (dis)continuity elements, reminding, and recognition, thus, are intimately connected in a complex equation.

TABLE 2.1
Connections Between Recall, Stanzas, and (Dis) Continuity Elements

Continuity Elements		
I. *Interactive wellformedness* Kinds: a. Assessments b. Formulations c. Sustainers d. Affirmations II. *Relative positioning of audience turns* a. Self-reminding prompts toward the beginning of narrative sequences b. Other-reminding prompts toward the beginning of narrative sequences	*Narrative wellformedness* Permits stanza segmentation	→ Recall
Discontinuity Elements		
I. *Interactive illformedness* Kinds: a. Extended pauses b. Repair II. *Relative positioning of audience turns* a. Other-reminding prompts toward the end of narrative sequences	*Narrative illformedness* Does not permit stanza segmentation	→ Reminding recognition

Table 2.1 is an attempt at clarifying connections between these terms. I need to note here, however, that my categorizing these terms into a table is by no means to suggest that distinctions and relationships between them are simple and clear-cut; I do so primarily for purposes of clarity. As we shall see, each of these terms informs others in multidimensional ways.

Connections between all of the preceding elements are relative. In some instances, patients engage successfully in recall, even when the interactions evidence discontinuity elements, just as there are instances in which patients are generally engaged in reminding/recognition while the interactions display continuity elements. Estimations and broad delineations between recall, reminding, recognition, and schematic processing that I make in the analysis, then, point to what seem generally evident in the data. A more important point that I hope to establish by exploring this complex web of connections is that these memory processes—for those of us who are "normal" as well as for those who have

AD—gain form in and through language and social interactions. They are grounded in a range of social dimensions including those of power and (in)equality as well as interactions that vary widely across audiences, settings, and time. Remembering, in the final analysis, is not an individual process but a social one.

3

Wellformedness in Alzheimer Interactions: Continuity Elements

> In planning our days and our lives we are composing the stories or the dramas we will act out and which will determine the focus of our attention and our endeavors, which will provide the principles for distinguishing foreground from background ... .We are constantly explaining ourselves to others. And finally each of us must count himself among his own audience since in explaining ourselves to others we are often trying to convince ourselves as well.
>
> —*David Carr* (1985)

The previous chapter looked at how stanzas allowed one to assess narrative wellformedness while certain kinds of continuity elements afforded insight into interactive wellformedness. In this chapter, I begin by considering how the narratives that Tina recounted to me at her home meet the wellformedness criteria established in this study. Her narratives and my interactions with her establish a kind of discourse yardstick by which to judge her talk in another setting (chap. 4) and with another audience (chap. 5). I then move into my larger data pool to examine how the positioning of particular utterances by both teller and audience in ongoing interactions serve different functions in the recalling process.

SOME NOTES ABOUT TINA

Before analyzing Tina's talk at home, I'd like to provide some ethnographic details about Tina's social world. These details provide a partial backdrop against which to locate her interactions with me and her husband, and serve as a contrast against which Ellie's social world and life story (chap. 6) can be understood.

I first met Tina, a white, middle-class woman, when I began working as a volunteer at the day-care center she attended. I worked at the center 2 days a week for a total of 10 hours weekly and had been there for 1 month before I recorded Tina. At the time of her recording, Tina was 65 years old. A few months earlier, she had taken a battery of tests including the minimental exam and the Boston naming test and was diagnosed to be in the mild to moderate stages of AD. (She demonstrated symptoms associated with this stage of the disease: short term memory loss, difficulty finding appropriate words, wandering attention.) She lived with her husband, N, in a residential part of suburban Los Angeles and seemed in very good care.

Tina comes across as an attractive woman with an exceptionally positive attitude. She had been a teacher of math and English before she was diagnosed with AD. She had been married once before, with two children from that marriage and one from her current marriage. She had spent a few years in India when N had been transferred there and expressed fond memories about her life abroad. She often confused me with one of her old Indian friends, frequently introducing me as her "friend from India" that she knew when she lived there. Because I actually am from India, we often had conversations about life and customs in that land. When Tina was about 64 years old, she started experiencing problems at school. Her husband suspected that all was not right when Tina started having trouble grading elementary math problems. On occasion, she also had gotten lost driving home from school. When she was diagnosed with AD, she gave up her job and began attending the day-care center where we met. She had been attending the center for about 7 months when I started to work there.

This day-care center is a nicely maintained and well-run establishment organized by a local church. Made up primarily of one very large room and two bathrooms, the center caters to both normal elderly and elderly with various kinds of impairments. At my time at the center, there were a total of 14 elderly on the roster: 8 were normal, 2 were AD patients (one of them being Tina), 2 had physical impairments and were in wheelchairs, 1 was recovering from a cerebral aneurism, and 1 from a stroke. Their ages ranged from 58 to 80.

The church associated with the center runs a seminary, and many of the students in the seminary work as interns at the center. Although these students have no formal training regarding caring for the elderly built into their curriculum, they do have occasional workshops with the manager of the center, who instructs them in activities that they use with the elderly. The manager herself has had training in gerontological-related issues and was at the time of my fieldwork in the process of conducting some research in gerontology. The activities that the elderly, including the AD patients, were generally engaged in appeared to be communicatively stimulating. These included watching and discussing old movies, discussing current political events, recounting personal experiences with particular holidays (meals they cooked for Thanksgiving or Christmas, family members they met during the holidays), all of which interested Tina, who was always very vocal. The elderly residents were also physically challenged: Occasionally, many who were physically able would go for a walk with a couple of the interns (Tina seldom stayed behind) while those in wheelchairs stayed behind and did some stretching exercises led by a supervisor.

Overall, the social and linguistic environment that Tina participated in, both at home and at the day-care center, appeared healthy and stimulating. She was engaged in communicative situations that facilitated her using language meaningfully both at home and at the day-care center, something that unfortunately some other AD patients that I worked with did not have (e.g., Ellie in chap. 6).

IDENTIFYING NARRATIVE SEQUENCES ACROSS THE DATA

Before we get into analyzing Tina's talk, a word about how I mark the beginnings and ends of narrative sequences across the data. I do so in terms of a co-occurrence of discourse features. I mark the beginnings of sequences by:

1. Statements that indicate the start of a new story on the part of the patient (e.g., "Let's see now ... " "Another thing occurred to me ... ", "You know, several years later I found ... ").
2. Topic changes (initiated by both patient and myself).
3. Speaker's tone ("beginnings" seem to be accompanied by an increased involvement and emphasis in the speaker's tone and/or an occasional lowering or raising of the speaker's voice).

I mark the ends of narrative sequences primarily in term of:

1. Pauses (at least 3 seconds long).
2. Falling intonation (marking closure).

3. Coda-like utterances in the Labovian sense (e.g., "so that was what happened ... " or "it didn't have to be that way y'know, but ... ").

WELLFORMEDNESS IN TINA'S TALK AT HOME

The following is the opening narrative sequence of my talk with Tina at home. (As the analyses in chaps. 4 and 5 point out, her talk with her husband and her talk [with me] at the day-care center do not evidence as much wellformedness.)

EXAMPLE 1
Stating the main point of the story
V: when you look back over your past Tina, what is it that stands out most?
T: ah { } well I guess the thing that stands out the most is   1
     ah my memories of my illness,
     and ah the fact that I couldn't even really walk.
     [...] and ah I

Support for the main point by focusing on an event
     daddy used to have to carry me and ah [...] you know   2
     it was a bad situation,
     but it brought us all close together.
     [...]

More detail about the event
     and ah you see   3
     they cut this wound on my back without anesthetic,
     [.] and I was just a teenager.
     and ah it was ah
     my mother didn't know they were going to operate on me.

Restating the main point
     and ah   4
     I kept deteriorating and deteriorating,
     and on,
     and I guess they felt they had to do something.

Restating stanza three: her mother's anger
     and I guess my mother was furious when she found   5
     out that they had cut this hole in my back,
     and ah
     [..]
V: what about other memories Tina?

Conclusion to the narrative despite my interruption. Restating points articulated in Stanza 2
     it was a painful situation.   6
     well, I have ah
     my my daddy used to carry me,
     and ah everywhere,
     and brought us really close together because aah,
     it was that kind of situation.
     [...]

This narrative segment lends itself to stanza segmentation in that each stanza takes a new perspective or introduces new information, thereby furthering the central idea introduced in Stanza 1. Stanza 1 sets up the central concern in her narrative, namely, her illness. She develops this concern in Stanzas 2 and 3, which deal with her operation ("Daddy used to have to carry me everywhere" "They cut a wound in my back without anesthetic"/"My mother didn't know they were going to operate on me"). Stanza 4 both justifies the need for the operation, a point she brings up in Stanza 3 ("I guess they felt they had to do something" because "I kept deteriorating and deteriorating"), and furthers the main point of her illness. Her points in Stanza 5 get tied up with points in Stanza 3 because she restates the same points ("My mother was furious when she found out that they had cut this hole in my back … "). Her line in the concluding stanza ("It was that kind of situation") echoes a point in Stanza 2 ("It was a bad situation"). Thus, by echoing previous ideas, the different lines in the stanzas "stitch the text together into a meaningful whole" (Gee, 1990, p. 189). Interestingly, Stanza 6 serves as her conclusion to her narrative, although I have initiated another turn. Tina does not respond to my question, "What about other memories Tina?" Instead, she goes on to complete her narrative by restating her opening points.

Stanzas in the preceding segment serve to unfold the information in her narrative incrementally: Each stanza develops both the structure and the topic of her narrative, and Tina is able to handle this in a sophisticated way. We see evidence of this in the following segment in which she talks about the time her husband fell seriously ill during their stay in India.

EXAMPLE 2
About how she went to India
T: Well ah [..] one day N came home and said "We are going to India
     for a few years."   43
     His boss wanted ah he wanted to set up something there and so we went,
     and we took our children.
V: Really

Preface to the event about her husband's illness
T: so they had the Indian experience which was good,   44
     and ah it was just a marvelous experience and time,
     but then of course at the end we had a very bad thing happen because
     my husband,
     ah contracted a thing called tropical sprew.

About tropical sprew as an illness
     and ah tropical sprew ah changes the stomach lining,   45
     and so all the food goes down faster,
     than it would normally do.

3. Wellformedness in Alzheimer Interactions

About how scared she was calling her mother
    [..] and so my husband,   46
    I looked at him one day and thought "I'm not going to be able to get him home,"
    and so ah my mother,
    I called my mother.

Her mother helping her
    my mother is in the travel agency,   47
    and she spends a lot of time just traveling around,
    and ah she said "we'll take him to Mayo Clinic."

N getting well
    Mayo clinic is a very fine clinic in the United States and,   48
    ah I think probably the best clinic and,
    so ah that's what we did we took him to Mayo clinic and we pulled him out.

Going back to N's illness
    but he was out,   49
    he was really,
    he had lost so much weight.

Going back to how scared she was
    it didn't dawn on me for a while,   50
    and then I looked at him one day and,
    I said "what's happened to him?
    he's just wasted away to nothing practically."
    it was awful.

Her mother's help and N getting well
    that day mother got him to the clinic,   51
    and right away they took care of him,
    so he pulled through it all right,
    thank goodness ah.

Contextualizing this event in her stay in India
    I loved India,   52
    still love India and always will love India,
    and ah but that was one thing that just scared me to death.
I: oh I should think it would
T: oh ya it was really frightening.

As with the earlier instance, we can see here how each stanza furthers the topic of the narrative. In Stanza 43, Tina tells me about how she went to India ("One day N came home and said 'We are going to India for a few years' ... and so we went") before introducing the fact of her husband's illness in Stanza 44 ("We had a very bad thing happen/because my husband ... contracted a thing called tropical sprew"). In Stanza 45 she steps out of her narrative to explain to me what tropical sprew is ("Tropical sprew ... changes the stomach lining/and so all the food goes down faster than it would normally do") before picking up the thread of her narrative again in Stanza 46. In Stanza 47 she talks about her mother's suggestion to take him to a clinic in the United States ("She said 'We'll take him to Mayo Clinic'"). Stanza 48, like Stanza 45, shows her once again stepping out of her narrative to explain to me why she and her mother decided to take N to the Mayo clinic ("Mayo clinic is a very fine clinic in the United States and/ah I think probably the best clinic ... "). In Stanza 49 we see her once again pick up the narrative thread by resuming her talk about N's illness ("He had lost so much weight"). Her ideas in Stanza 50 ("It was awful") are reiterations of her ideas at the start of her narrative ("We had a very bad thing happen," Stanza 44). Likewise, her ideas in Stanza 51 ("That day mother got him to the clinic ... and he pulled through all right") reiterate her previously mentioned ideas in Stanzas 47 ("Mother ... said 'we'll take him to Mayo Clinic'") and 48 ("we pulled him out ..."). This echoing of previous ideas serves as a preface for her concluding stanza (#52) where she recontextualizes the event as something that occurred during her stay in India.

Thus, (the structures of) both illness narratives lend themselves to stanza segmentation. She is able to talk at considerable length in both, providing details to support her points. We also are able to see the thematic development of her central points—about her near death in the first one, and her husband's near death in the second—in the continuity between the ideas that make up the stanzas, as well as between the stanzas themselves. Both structurally and thematically, then, the preceding narratives meet the wellformedness criteria.

Tina's narratives about her marriages—recorded as well in her interaction with me at home—are also wellformed. In the following segment she talks about her present marriage to N. Until this point, she has been talking about her previous unhappy marriage to M, and why she thinks things went wrong.

EXAMPLE 3
V: What has your marriage to N been like?
Comparing her present marriage to her previous one:
T: It's been good, really, 32
no not in this one.
I'm glad because I had so much before with M,
so much problems.

Justification for divorcing M
well it took me a while to get the courage to get the divorce, 33
but I did I did,
and ah it worked out much better.
[...]

Not trusting M with her children
and I was worried when I was with M, 34

was worried about the children,
because I didn't exactly trust Marks.

Not trusting M's character
and he was so,   35
he didn't seem,
he was not a sincere person,
and if you are not sincere,
you are not good for much.

Comparing her previous marriage to the present one
so [..] with N our marriage was very happy,   36
and it was very good for the children too [..].
V: did they adapt to that/were you ever afraid
that they would not adapt to N?
T: ah they/ah no,
I wasn't,
I wasn't because they liked him right off the bat.
V: oh ya?
T: ya
V: its hard not to.

Justification for why her marriage to N is happy
T: ya, it was really wonderful because the children,   37
when I introduced N to the children,
he picked them up you know,
he was instantly into the picture.

Support for Stanza 37
and ah he's been a wonderful father to them,   38
[.] I can't imagine him being anything else,
he is such a loving person,
a very warm person [...].

Repeating points of Stanza 37
and ah when I introduced the children to him,   39
he picked them up,
and ah it was wonderful.

Comparing N to M/similar to Stanza 36
I never thought I'd get so embroiled in a situation as I did with Bob Marks,
he was really the antithesis of ah ah ah [...].   40
V: N

Conclusion
T: right N.   41
get my husbands mixed up,
so its been a very very happy family,
alls well that ends well,
[...]

The stanzas in the this segment, like those discussed previously, unfold information incrementally. Each stanza deals with a particular perspective on a character, action, event, or claim, leading the narrative up to its high point ("He was really the antithesis of N"). All the information that Tina provides in the course of her narrative builds semantically on previously introduced information.

In Stanza 32 she lays the groundwork for what her narrative is about, namely her unhappy marriage to M and her present, happy marriage to N ("N not in this one.... I'm glad because I had so much before/with M/so much problems"). In Stanza 33, she justifies her need to divorce M ("It worked out so much better"), whereas in Stanzas 34 and 35 she goes into detail as to why her relationship with him did not work ("I was worried about the children" ... "he was not a sincere person"). Stanza 37, in which she talks about her children taking to N ("When I introduced N to the children/he picked them up you know/he was instantly into the picture ... "), gets tied up to Stanza 34 in which she had voiced her distrust of M with the children ("I was worried about the children/because I didn't exactly trust M"). In Stanzas 38 and 39 she provides more detail about N and her children ("And ah he's been a wonderful father to them/he is such a loving person/he picked them up/ah it was wonderful"), whereas Stanza 40 ("I never thought I'd get so embroiled in a situation/as I did with M") reiterates ideas of Stanza 34 ("And I was worried when I was with M"), thereby tying them all together. Finally in Stanza 41, she brings the whole story to a close ("It's been a very very happy family/all's well that ends well").

Her narrative about her previous marriage evidences such segmentation as well.

EXAMPLE 4
T: he may have had other relationships and stuff,
V: did he ever say so?

Introducing her unhappy marriage
T: he didn't ever say so,   21
   but I think I was sure that he did,
   so we got the divorce finally.

Justification for divorce
   ya it just went on too long and it wasn't pleasant,   22
   and I had the children too to take care of,
   so we came to a parting of the ways.

More justification
   and it was better that way,   23
   than to let the whole thing start to deteriorate,
   and with the children knowing that it wasn't a happy household,
   and so N and I got married.
V: how long after that?

Comparing N with previous husband
T: it wasn't too long,   24

>   I'd say about 3 years,
>   [.] and ah N was just ah,
>   the ah [..] the opposite of this man,
>   and ah I was very lucky that he wanted to marry me.
>
> *Introducing the kind of man N is*
>   I thought probably that some men would not want to,   25
>   have a ah have me because it is sort of like [.],
>   used [laughs] merchandise you know.
>
> *Conclusion*
>   and ah I never had that feeling,   26
>   because N was a very honorable person,
>   and still is […].

As with the earlier narrative, we can see that stanzas operate to structure her ideas. In Stanza 21 she responds to my question about her marriage being unhappy because he had relationships with other women ("I was sure that he did/so we got the divorce finally"), whereas in Stanzas 22 and 23 she provides justification for the divorce ("It wasn't pleasant/I had the children too to take care of/it was better that way/than to let the whole thing start to deteriorate/and with the children knowing that it wasn't a happy household"). At the end of Stanza 23 she brings up the idea of how she and N got married, and from this point on her stanzas (24 to 26) are about N. However, she is careful to establish connections between her first husband and N; she does this by contrasting them: ("N was just … the opposite of this man/and ah I was very lucky that he wanted to marry me/N was a very honorable person, and still is").

PERCENTAGE OF CONNECTED SPEECH IN TINA'S TALK AT HOME

The preceding four narratives, all of which meet the narrative wellformedness criteria for this study (i.e., they all lend themselves to stanza segmentation, demonstrating that Tina's is connected and continuous), show how I am able to engage Tina in recall at home. Of course, one reason I am able to do so is because her talk is connected enough to permit such segmentation. Toward gauging what percentage of her total speech at home is continuous, I parsed her talk into segments made up of at least three connected lines (see Table 3.1).

TABLE 3.1
Percentage of Connected Speech in Tina's Talk at Home

Percentage of 3-Line Segments Drawn Out of a Total of 384 Lines
93%

From a total of 384 lines that comprised Tina's talk, 357 lines lent themselves to this method of segmentation. This means that 93% of her talk lent itself to 3-line segments. As we see in parts of chapters 4 and 5, her talk with her husband and with me at the day-care center do not evidence such connectedness.

Continuity Elements in Our Interaction

One reason why Tina's narratives at home are as connected and continuous as they are is partly because our interaction has several (more) continuity elements (than discontinuity elements) that serve both to faciliate recall and to keep our talk on track. Although there are discontinuity elements (chap. 4 goes into detail about this), these are by no means a predominant feature in the interaction (as they are in other instances)

Newsmarks in our interaction. Newsmarks, as discussed earlier, emphasize the prior turn's noteworthiness or surprise value for the recipient. They usually lead to further talk, either by the teller of the news or by the audience, thus maintaining continuity in the interaction. The following instances from my interaction with Tina (my newsmarks are italicized) at home demonstrate this:

EXAMPLE 5
```
        she was a very strong woman
        she just recently died [says this softly]
V:      really?
T:      uh huh [ ... .]
        but she was oh,
        it was one of those things ....
```

EXAMPLE 6
```
V:      so did she continue to work in the laboratory
        after your father died?
T:      ya
V:      really?
T:      and ah she,
        its just been recently that she died,
        that was such a shock to me....
```

EXAMPLE 7
```
V:      did they adapt to that/ were you ever afraid
        that they would not adapt to Nick?
T:      ah they ah no,
        I wasn't,
        I wasn't because they liked him right off the bat.
```

V: oh ya?
T: ya
V: it's hard not to....

EXAMPLE 8
V: what do you think about marriage Tina?
T: Oh, I think it is the way to go really.
V: *ya? you believe in it?*
T: ya, yes I do ...

In Examples 5 and 6 Tina talks about her mother. In Example 5 she says of her mother, "She was a very strong woman/she just recently died," to which I respond with a "Really?", implying thereby that I found her information newsworthy. I respond with "really" again in Example 6 when she tells me about her mother working in the laboratory. In both cases, my responses serve to further our interaction by eliciting more talk from Tina; they also serve to keep our interaction on the track (topic) of her mother ("It's just been recently that she died/that was such a shock to me"). In Examples 7 and 8 my newsmarks "Oh ya?" and "Ya? You believe in it" seem to serve the same function.

Formulations in Our Talk at Home. Formulations on my part serve to keep our talk continuous and connected in that they exhibit an understanding of what is important to focus on, clarify, or confirm in the prior turn(s). We see evidence of this in segments such as the following.

EXAMPLE 9
V: when you look back over your past Tina, what is it that stands out most?
T: ah { } well I guess the thing that stands out the most is,
   ah my memories of my illness.
V: really?
T: and ah the fact that I couldn't even really walk.
V: how old were you?
T: oh let's see
   I was in Kindergarten
V: *ya, you were really young*
T: uh huh

EXAMPLE 10
V: had you kept in touch with him at all?
T: no
V: so after the divorce you never met him or any
   thing?
T: no, we don't go in the same circles because,
   our friends aren't the same or anything.
V: *so he never kept in touch with the children or anything?*
T: no [..] in fact at one time I had to have the fight the [..] the [..],
   [searching for words]

        he didn't keep up with his child care support,
        and ah I had to get the law after him,
        because the children couldn't have been supported.
V: *that couldn't have been easy*
T: no it wasn't....

EXAMPLE 11
V: so did she continue to work in the laboratory after your father died?
T: ya
V: really?
T: and ah she its just been recently that she died,
       that was such a shock to me,
       somehow I felt my mother would never die,
V: *I know what you mean/there are certain fixtures in your life that*
       you think will never go
T: yes uhuh ya I just couldn't believe it,
       when my sister said "I have something to tell you and it is going to be hard,
       for you to take" and ah "you know mother died last night,"
       and ah that was very hard to take [tears in her eyes].

Nofsinger (1991) pointed out that formulations can occur either as an immediate response to a prior utterance or as a delayed summary of a prior stretch of talk. In Example 9 my utterance, "Ya you were really young" occurs as an immediate response to Tina's prior utterance about her illness when she was in kindergarten. However, my formulation in Example 10 occurs after Tina's extended turn. In the previous stanza, she has been talking about the hard time she had with her first husband and how she had "to get the law after him." My formulation, "That couldn't have been easy," serves both to summarize what she has been saying and communicate sympathy with her position. In Example 11 we see that two of my three utterances are continuity elements: "Really" serves as a newsmark to confirm an earlier utterance (about her mother working in the laboratory after her father died), whereas "I know/there are certain fixtures ... you think will never go" serves to empathize with Tina's sentiments about not being able to accept the death of some people. Continuity in the representative segments just discussed is achieved because my turns display my understanding of the gist of Tina's talk. My ability to extrapolate the main point of what she is saying serves to elicit more talk from her, thereby furthering our interaction.

Affirmations in Our Interaction.   Similar to formulations are continuity devices that I refer to as *affirmations*. Unlike formulations, affirming utterances do not demonstrate a summary of prior talk; instead, they display agreement. The following segments from our interaction at home illustrate this.

3. Wellformedness in Alzheimer Interactions

EXAMPLE 12
T: when my sister said "I have something to tell you,
and it is going to be hard for you to take,"
and ah "you know mother died last night,"
and ah that was very hard to take {tears in her eyes}.
I think with everybody's mother,
that their mothers are such important persons.
V: (*softly*) *very much so Tina/specially if you are very close*
T: and we were very close,
well both my daddy and mother were very close to me.

EXAMPLE 13
T: I say to myself,
"you can't have your mother all of the time,"
and ah but ah,
and I did see a lot of my mother,
and I adored my mother,
and ah she was a wonderful person.
V: *I'm sure*
you said she was very strong
T: oh yes.

EXAMPLE 14
V: did they adapt to that/were you ever afraid that they would not adapt to N?
T: ah they/ ah no
I wasn't,
I wasn't because they liked him right off the bat.
V: oh ya?
T: ya
V: *it's hard not to*
T: ya, it was really wonderful because the children....

In all of the preceding instances my italicized utterances display agreement with Tina's prior stretch of talk. In Example 12, she talks about how hard her mother's death was for her and concludes her turn by saying; "I think with everybody's mother/that their mothers are such important persons." My affirmative response to that: "Very much so Tina/specially if you are very close" serves to both acknowledge Tina's sentiments and further her talk. We see that she, in turn, affirms my utterance ("especially if you are very close") by restating it ("And we were very close") in her next turn. We see this in Examples 13 and 14 as well. In Example 13 my utterance ("I'm sure") displays agreement with Tina's talk about her mother's qualities ("She was a wonderful woman"), whereas, my utterance in Example 14 ("It's hard not to") displays my understanding of why Tina's children adapted to N so easily; it evidences my agreement with Tina about the kind of person N is.

TABLE 3.2
Percentage of Some Continuity Elements in Tina's Interactions With Me at Home, at the Day-Care Center and With Her Husband

Continuity Elements	Home (%)	Day-Care (%)	Husband (%)
Newsmarks	8.75	1.6	0
Fomulations	15.46	1.6	0.7
Affirmations	6.51	2.2	1.77
Sustainers/evaluations	4.27	0	0
Total	34.99	5.4	2.47

Percentage of Continuity Devices in the Different Interactions. These representative segments illustrate some ways in which continuity elements sustain our interaction. To gain a better sense of how my role as recipient contributes to maintaining continuity in our interaction Table 3.2 presents a percentage form a breakdown of some of continuity elements my turns constituted. Recipient turns in this interaction total 54. As a way of contrasting how these fare against my turns in our interaction at the day-care center and in Tina's interaction with her husband, I present those relevant numbers as well.

Almost 35% of recipient turns in my interaction with Tina at home are continuity elements, almost 7 times more than my continuity utterances at the day-care center and almost 15 times more than N's utterances.

I also attempted to get a breakdown of how these continuity elements operated in my interactions with the other 15 patients. All of these patients were recorded in settings in which they were most comfortable. In some cases these settings constituted their homes in which they were cared for by family members, in others retirement communities or day-care centers where patients spent most of their time. In many cases, the time at the day-care centers afforded these patients the most linguistic and communicative chances they got in a day. Most of them were driven back to their apartments or homes after their time in center was over, where they were often visited by a social worker who would check in on them late in the evening to make sure they were settled for the night Table 3.3 lays out the number of continuity elements in my interactions with them. Unlike Tina's case, these patients were not recorded across settings.

Of all my turns in these interactions, 59.2% are continuity elements that both facilitate recall from the patient and maintain continuity in the interaction. However, as we see in chapter 4, there are certain moves I make

3. Wellformedness in Alzheimer Interactions

TABLE 3.3
Percentage of Some Continuity Elements in My Interactions
With all 16 Patients in Settings Where They Were Comfortable

Continuity Elements	Across All 16 Interactions
Newsmarks	11.01
Formulations	16.06
Affirmations	20.00
Sustainers	12.05
Total	59.21

that inhibit the patients' ability to engage in extended and meaningful talk, thus rendering our interaction(s) discontinuous.

Interactive Wellformedness: Positioning of Audience Turns

Like continuity elements, the *positioning* of certain turns in narrative sequences, by both teller and audience, seems to play a role in whether the patient is engaged in recall. I mentioned earlier that as audience and researcher I tried to get the patients to engage in extended turns. At several points this meant attempting to convert their reminding process (wherein they did not engage in a narrative turn) to recall where in they did.

The data reveal two kinds of reminding prompts: *self-prompted reminding*, in which the patients' current talk reminds them of another life event, and *other-prompted reminding*, in which an audience prompt reminds the teller of a related life event. Examples 15 and 16 illustrate both kinds, respectively.

EXAMPLE 15
Self-prompted reminding
D: let me try and see what is her name?   1
    I can't remember it ah   2
    I believe it's Sandy; that's right   3
    [...]

EXAMPLE 2
Other-prompted reminding
A: and so I tried y'know   1
    it was hard and ah am ahh I ah   2
V: you were saying that you tried to?   3
A: ah am ah ...

In Line 1 of Example 15, Diane tries to prompt herself into remembering the name of the person she is talking about and in Line 3 is able to come up with it ("I believe it's Sandy, that's right"). In Example 16, however, I am the one trying to prompt Amelia into remembering something (Line 3) when she seems to lose track of what she was saying (Line 2).

Self-Reminding Prompts Toward the Beginning of Narrative Sequences

EXAMPLE 17

V: uhm how did you meet your husband?
D: *let's see now how did I meet him I have to stop and think*
it was George Foster.
V: hmmm
D: and he came from Canada to visit some relatives,   1
that I know,
they had a daughter my age,
but he didn't seem to shine up to her for some reason.
uhm.
V: mm
D: *let me try and see what was her name?*

    I can't remember her name right now,   2
    uh gosh, well it doesn't matter about her name,

    he came down,   3
    and … well, these people wanted me to meet him.

    or he wanted to meet someone in Connecticut,   4
    and of course I was very friendly with the daughter.

    and the rest of the family,   5
    but especially the girls,
    we went out together.
V: mmm

D: so that was how I met him,   6
came down from there to visit these people,
and he never went back to Massachussets.
V: I see I see

D: ya he never went back,   7
let's see now he liked what he saw down here you know,
and the people were friendly with him,
and well, we just got very close and then finally married.

    he wanted me to go back with him,   8
    but I would not go if I we were not married,
    so he says "I'm going to stay here until y-,
    I can bring you back.

	and I had friends from there, and I knew they were very friendly.	9
	so I went back, and by golly I got such a greeting you know, it was really wonderful....	10

When in Line 1 I ask Diana how she met her husband, her response "Let's see now, how did I meet him, I have to think" (Line 2) is a self-reminding prompt that successfully triggers her recalling details about when and how she met George Foster. We see her prompt herself again a few lines later just before the beginning of Stanza 2 ("Let me try and see what was her name?"). In both instances, Diana is able to pick up the threads of her thought and continue with her recalling process.

Another segment in which a patient's self-reminding prompt at the beginning of a narrative sequence does not impede recall is the following.

EXAMPLE 4

V:	what about college did you go to college?	
K:	I went to college for I think oh about 2 years, and then I had to change my uh set up because uh I don't remember, who it was, whether it was my mother or my father, needed uh a lot of doctoring. *let me see* *I think it was ah ah my father.*	1
V:	oh really?	
K:	yeah So I had to quit my job,	2
V:	uhhumm	
K:	and help	
V:	with the medical bills?	
K:	help pay *I think [...] it was my mother* *but I I'm not sure [...]* Maybe it was my father	3
V:	ya	
K:	but those things don't stay with me, Soon we were out of the woods and and uh everything, was under control, and the doctor assured me that we don't have anything to worry, out I went.	4
	when I helped them, when my mother or my father was ill, I, I stayed there.	5
	I left my own house, and I stayed there with them, to help them.	6

V:	I see	
K:	But when they were under control, I left,	7
V:	I see so you'd already been living outside your	
K:	yes	
V:	your parents' house, the place you grew up?	
K:	uhhuh.	

We see in this instance that Kasper's self-reminding prompt occurs toward the beginning of his narrative sequence (within the first three stanzas) and that it does not impede his recalling process. His first self-reminding prompt, "Let me see, I think it was my father," is followed by details about his quitting his job. Likewise, he continues talking about his parent's illness after his second relatively indirect self-reminding prompt wherein he pauses first for 4 seconds ("I think [….] it was my mother") and then again for 5 seconds ("But I'm not sure { ….}").

Examples 17 and 18 indicate that the patients are able to sustain their recalling process when their self-reminding prompts occur at the beginning of narrative segments. To get a sense of how systematically this occurred through the data, I computed the average number of self-reminding prompts in one interaction, which was 3, with the average number of narrative sequences per interaction, which was 8. This meant that 37% of self-reminding prompts at the beginning of narrative segments did not inhibit the teller's recalling process.

Self-Reminding Prompts Toward the End of Narrative Sequences

EXAMPLE 19

F:	I worked in an electronics company.	
V:	uhhuhmm	
F:	and I was so deeply involved,	1
	day and night that I felt whatever I need,	
	I'll catch up while I'm on the way,	
	but uh I didn't.	
	I didn't make a point of anything in particular,	2
	so that I was able to hold my own with the customer,	
	as well as with my boss.	
	and uh that sufficed for that was ok,	3
	that was good,	
	that was a good job.	
	[…]	
V:	uhhuhmm	
	so you were there for a long time?	

V:	did you do different things for them?	
F:	No I didn't do anything different that that,	4
	uh I don't remember how long ago this was,	
	my memory is playing terrible tricks on me.	
V:	is it?	
F:	I had a memory that if you open a book and you see the word,	5
	well I got to the point where I didn't have to open the book,	
	and I didn't have to study it.	
	I didn't,	6
	I could retain it,	
	I could grasp it,	
	I could I could be on my own for whatever,	
	That was a wonderful time [....]	
	let's see where was I?	7
F:	Uh when we were in a meeting,	
	and when then when the man in charge uh started,	
	"you do this, why didn't you do that and how about that?"	
	It came to me,	
	I didn't give him a chance to to say 'how about that?'	
	I unfold the whole thing,	8
	cause I knew that somewhere along the line I would be in in,	
	that same sw switch,	
	Uh, "what did you do and what the hell is matter with you?"	
	You know things like that.	
	They were a good company,	9
	and they were they did a good job,	
	and they were worthwhile working for,	
	But after a while it got to a point where I was doing the same thing today, yesterday, tomorrow, next week.	
	and so I started to look elsewhere,	10
	They were sorry to leave, for me to leave.	
V:	I bet they were	
	and uh I sensed that they're going to increase my salary in order to retain me,	
	but I wouldn't I wouldn't uh accept it,	11
	I would explain to them why, what and how,	
	"you're you're a fine company" and begin with that,	
	Well I wanted to go into a different field a better field,	
	and and uh I it ah it stood me in good stead.	

From Stanzas 1 to 7 we see Frank recalling details about his job. The end of Stanza 6 appears to mark the end of that narrative sequence: His utterance, "That was a wonderful time," is spoken with a falling intonation marking closure, and it is followed by a 4-second pause that seems to indicate that he has finished saying what he wants to about that topic. However, after the pause, at the begining of Stanza 7 we see him prompt himself with "Let's see, where was I?" and we see him getting started on another narrative sequence. The following segment illustrates this as well.

EXAMPLE 20

L: you see my uncle was a sea captain,   1
so I knew all the goings on,
and that ship went out.

and I saw the ship go,   2
and it went to Boston,
and it had passengers on it.

and the people won't believe it,   3
but you see, it was ah,
it was one of the very first vessels to have a double bottom.

And today I guess of all passenger vessels,   4
that 90 90 percent are double-bottomed,
just be not because of that one.

but there were quite a few,
ahhh eh uh I don't know what you want to call,
but the wreckages,
and the boat get on rocks and bad navigation and that sort of thing,

and if they have a double bottom they'll float along.   5

And just hope that they don't go on at high tide,   6
because if they go at high tide they're much worse off,
than if they go at low tide,
because you float off.

And I've heard people go and remark after my telling 'em,   7
I've heard about that the other people did,
"Well he didn't know much about it,
he was too young, a child" and oh.

It's just that I was exposed to all that,   8
and for heaven sakes if you are and that's very important,
thing in your life if you remember it.

V: ya you would remember things like that, I know.

L: And that ship went to Boston,   9
it went back with the passengers,
which today would not be allowed,
Soo:[…] let me think   10
what was I saying?
oh yes about traveling on the boat.

if the weather is beautiful, it's fine,   11
if the weather is rough it's miserable,
and it can be very rough going from Boston to Yama.

	and of course the sea boats today are much better,	12
	but even so they are still boats going on a rough journey.	
V:	uhhuh	

L:	But it's well,	13
	they used to leave Boston late in the afternoon,	
	and make that crossing from Boston to Yama so that uh,	
	they're there very early in the morning.	

	That's one of the reasons why they go to Yama in day light,	14
	'cause because the harbor is very winding and has high tide, (laughs)	
	and you can go on the rocks,	
	and we did,	15
	and the ship had a double bottom,	
	and we went back to Boston that night with my great greater.	

| | great great I don't know how many greats there were in there, | 16 |
| | but he was the sea captain [...]. | |

L in this segment starts off by talking about his uncle who was a sea captain, and he devotes Stanzas 1 though 9 to double-bottomed boats. He appears to mark the end of that narrative with a 4-second pause as well as a coda-like utterance about the ship that was not double-bottomed going back to Boston. At the beginning of Stanza 10, we see him prompting himself with "Let me think, what was I saying?" and continue his recalling process, with his focus this time on traveling by boat from Boston to Yama.

Once again to get a sense of how systematically this occurred through the data, I attempted to figure out what percentage of these turns facilitated recall. There are an average of 5 self-reminding prompts (toward the end of narrative sequences) out of an average of 8 narrative sequences per interaction. This means that 62.5% of self-reminding prompts at the end of narrative sequences seem to facilitate recall. Table 3.4 lays this out along with the percentage of self-reminding prompts toward the beginning of narrative sequences.

It appears, then, that when patients prompt themselves toward the end of narrative sequences, they are more likely to get back into the recalling mode as opposed to when they prompt themselves toward the beginning of their narratives. It is likely that patients are able to continue the recalling

TABLE 3.4
Position of Patient Moves That Seem to Facilitate Recall

Self-Reminding Prompts at Beginning of Narrative Segments (%)	*Self-Reminding Prompts Toward the End of Narrative Segments (%)*
37	62.5

process because they have "warmed up" and have figured out the activity in which I, as audience, am attempting to engage them. In other words, they seem to have unconsciously realized that I want them to recall and engage in extensive turns.

We also saw how the patients' ability to engage in recall depends simultaneously on kinds of continuity elements that the audience makes to keep the interaction afloat (e.g., as in Tina's case).

4

Narrative and Interactive Illformedness in Alzheimer Talk

> Although narration moves inescapably backward in its concern with the understanding of the past-in-the-present, the view of development that derives from it can retain a focus on the forward movement that is rendered in the texts provided. Thus perhaps, paradoxically, it is out of retrospection that a project, an approximation toward desired ends, can be revealed. The shape that emerges out of the past extends itself into the future. It is this temporal dialogue which can lay the foundation for a new conceptualization of life-span developmental knowledge.
>
> —*Mark Freeman* (1984)

The previous chapter discussed ways in which Tina's talk at home was extended and meaningful enough to allow stanza segmentation. We also examined how her ability to produce wellformed talk is partially a result of particular kinds, as well as specific positioning, of audience moves that keeps the interaction relatively smooth and on track. In this chapter, I call attention to some interactional features that inhibit Tina's efforts to successfully engage in recall at the day-care center. As with the previous chapter, I also point out how the positioning of other reminding turns at certain points in the interactions renders both patient talk and interactions discontinuous and illformed.

TINA'S INABILITY TO NARRATE AT THE DAY-CARE CENTER

Evident in the transcripts as well as in the segments to be presented is that much of Tina's talk at the day-care center remains at the level of conversation. The opening segment of her talk is one (extreme) example in which Tina is not able to narrate.

EXAMPLE 1
V: Tell me about yourself Tina.
T: oh I have,   1
   I am one of three sisters and ah,
   ah no brothers unfortunately,
   and ah we always wanted brothers, [V: did you}
   and we didn't have any.
   [...]

V: where are your sisters now?
T: well one sister is in ah,   2
   oh she is off.
   off off [..].
V: is she out of town?
T: she is ah [...].   3

V: what's her name?
T: her name is Barbara Lee[..],   4

V: is she older than you?
T: yes, uh huh [....].   5

V: do you have other sisters?
T: Barbara Lee is an ah is she [...].   6

V: what about Margaret Ann/I think you once
   mentioned that you had a sister.
   called Margaret?   7
T: yes Margaret, yes [....].
V: so there are three of you?
T: yes, I think that's right.

None of Tina's utterances here—"she is off," "she is ah [...]," "her name is Barbara Lee [..]," "yes, uh huh [....]"—develop into stanzas. (The numbers next to the utterances point to potential openings for stanza development.) Given that stanzas enable us to see how information in a narrative is unpackaged in small increments of topically related units, we can see that the utterances in the preceding segment are not continuous enough to permit such parsing, largely because there is not enough new information. Because this is the opening segment of our interaction, it could be argued, of course, that the reason Tina does not narrate is because she has not yet grasped the nature of the activity in which we are engaged, that she has not figured out that my prompts are cues for her to talk extensively. But this cannot account for other instances in our interaction in which she demonstrates a similar tendency. Take, for instance, the following segment where we talk about her trip abroad.

> EXAMPLE 2
> V: Why did you go to India, Tina? 26
>
> T: I had always wanted to go to India,
> I had always been interested in India,
> one day my ah daddy came home and said "we are going to India,"
> and my first reaction was "oh a terrible place," 27
> that dirty place/ you'll get sick all the time."
>
> and my mother said "you must go, 28
> it is so fascinating" and so we went,
> I wouldn't have given it up for anything.
>
> V: so you and your husband went? 29
> T: Ya.
> Did you enjoy your stay there?
> T: oh ya.
> I had always wanted to go to India.
>
> V: Is there any event that stands out,
> in your memory about your stay there? 30
> T: [...]
>
> V: can you recall any event about India,
> Tina? 31
> T: we stayed in the hills,
> it was beautiful and fascinating.
>
> V: Tell me about one incident during
> your stay there. 32
> T: it was beautiful [...].

As with the earlier instance, we see that Tina's talk here does not allow stanza parsing. Her talk starts off as a narrative (Stanzas 26 to 28) in which she talks about how her trip to India came about ("I had always wanted to go to India ... and my first reaction was 'oh a terrible place'/ I wouldn't have given it up for anything"), but she does not sustain her effort. In fact, in some instances, she does not respond at all. In Stanza 29, for instance, she does not pick up my prompts as cues for her to keep talking ("So you and your husband went"/"did you enjoy your stay there?"); in Stanza 30 she is unresponsive to my cue ("Is there any event that stands out in your memory about your stay there?"). In Stanzas 31 and 32 we see her responding to my questions ("We stayed in the hills/it was beautiful and fascinating ... /it was beautiful [...]"), but, once again, she does not develop her utterances into narratives. Hutchinson and Jensen (1980) suggest that this inability to provide elaborate responses to questions may have to do with a reduction in the number of functioning neurons in the patient's central nervous system.

I do not mean to imply that Tina is unable to narrate at the center. She does narrate, but she needs more prompting than she did in our interaction at her home. Take, for instance, the following piece where she is describing her father's funeral.

EXAMPLE 3

V: how old were you?
T: ah […] I'd say seven or so,   44
   and ah [..] when daddy died I didn't believe it,
   didn't believe it was real,
   that he died and ah [….].

   and ah I said I wanted to go to,   45
   the funeral,
   I insisted and pretty soon my mother gave in,
   and ah but she was right,
   because we got to the funeral,
   an ah [… …] ah [… ..] ah [… .] ah […].

V: What happened at the funeral?   46
T: ah she said ah,
   she didn't want me to go to the funeral,
   and I insisted and ah she,
   until then ah she knew I was upset,
   and she didn't want to make too much of it and ah she,
   […]

V: what happened then?   47
T: and so [… …] ah
   when they had an open casket sometimes,
   they have a closed casket,
   they had an open casket for daddy.

   and ah [..] when I saw him,   48
   I ah ah got very upset and said,
   "not my daddy, he's not my daddy,"
   'cause he was you know,
   he was so cold in the casket.

   and ah I did never see him that way,   49
   because he seemed such a warm hearted person,
   and ah he was such a wonderful person and ah,
   I started screaming so they had to take me out and,
   ah [..] that was the last I saw of him […].

In Stanza 44 we see Tina lay out the gist of her narrative: that as a child she had not been able to accept her father's death and that she did not believe "it was real." In Stanza 45 she goes into how her mother did not want her to go to the funeral and how Tina insisted ("I said I wanted to go to the funeral/I insisted and pretty soon my mother gave in"). At the end of that stanza we see her voice trail off (ah [……] ah ah […..] ah [….] ah […]). As a way of getting her back into her narrative, I prompt her with "What happened at the funeral?" but instead of continuing her narrative from where she left off, she repeats, in response, the points of Stanza 45 ("She didn't want me to go to the funeral/and I insisted and/she knew I was upset/and she didn't want to make too much of it"). She has to be prompted again with "What happened then?" in order for her to complete her narrative.

Although Tina's narrative does reach its high point ("When I saw him/I ah ah got very upset and said/'not my daddy, he's not my daddy'"), it does so only with recipient help. In other words, her narrative needs to be *scaffolded* in order for it to be complete and coherent. As we saw, her narratives at home did not demonstrate this need for scaffolding; Tina is able to bear the onus of narrating by herself.

EVIDENCE OF INCOHERENCE IN HER SPEECH

Also evident in her talk at the day-care center are lapses in coherence. In the following segment she narrates about her marriage, when all of a sudden her talk ceases to make sense.

EXAMPLE 4
V: tell me about your marriage Tina? 13
T: oh, I've oh my husband works for the
Industrial Relations,
for Cal Tech Industrial Relations, 14
and ah he's a busy busy guy [laughs].
[..]
V: How did you meet him? 15
T: I met him with some friends and ah ah [..],
we got to talking about things,
and we just sort of escalated.

V: how old were you? 16
T: oh I was not a youngster at that particular point in time,
but he is always very busy,
he works for Cal Tech.

> but we see a lot of each other too, 17
> we see to that,
> I don't want a marriage where you are always away from your husband,
> it's not a good way to be at it.
> [...]
>
> takes two for a marriage it does, 18
> but by the same token both parties have to fight it,
> I mean they have to struggle make it right,
> and my husband is very busy,
> and ahm ah sometimes away a lot [.] from home.
>
> but tt [] it was something that you do, 19
> *and then it's you hop up and say hey look here I am,*
> *I'm already comin up* [ ].
> {gets distracted, addresses another AD (severe) patient} *did you drop somebody?*
> *oh good* [....]

Tina's talk in the this segment, although not extensively developed into a narrative (the way her talk at home is), starts off wellformed inasmuch as her utterances are topically related. She begins by talking about where her husband works ("My husband works for the Industrial Relations/for Cal Tech Industrial Relations") and about where she met him ("I met him with some friends"). She also implies that her husband's busy life does not permit them to spend much time together ("But he is always very busy ..."). She articulates her views about this and about marriage in general in Stanzas 17 and 18 ("but we see a lot of each other too/we see to that/I don't want a marriage where you are always away from your husband/it's not a good way to be at it"). Meaningful up until this point, Tina's talk suddenly becomes incoherent in Stanza 19 ("But tt [] it was something that you do/and then it's you hop up and say hey look here I am/I'm already comin up ... did you drop somebody? oh good" [.]). And yet not all of Stanza 19 is incoherent: The first line of this stanza can in fact be seen as topically related to her utterances in the previous stanza ("My husband ... is away a lot ... from home/but ... it was something that you do"). But the rest of her lines in this stanza do not make any sense, at least not in the light of her previous utterances. Bloom, Rocisano, & Heed (1979) maintained that senile people, like children, are likely to get distracted easily by things in their immediate environment. It is possible that Tina has lost her train of thought because other directives "transitorily entered [her] immediate consciousness" (Hutchinson & Jensen, 1980, p. 71).

EVIDENCE OF EGOCENTRIC SPEECH

We also see evidence of egocentric speech in her talk at the day-care center. In the following segment she talks about her children. Although some of the utterances in this segment are clear, others are not. Actually, on the face of it, these unclear utterances seem disconnected and incoherent. However, these "incoherent" utterances can be seen to make sense if we understand them in terms of information Tina has established much earlier in our interaction.

EXAMPLE 5
V: did you have any children?   20
T: Ya, three
   Ya Mike, Didi and Vicki and Jerry and Trevor and Elise,
V: really?
   are they all your children or your grandchildren too?
T: grandchildren too.
V: where are they? are they in LA?

T: well ah ah well yes,   21
   Vicki and Jerry and Didi and N and I,
   and N my husband and,
   ah his last name is Nichols.

   and ah ah he he always goes by N,   22
   but the children don't go by N,
   they call him Dad.
   [..] and I like it that way [..].
   I mean not had a father other than the father I lost in the war,
   ah I like it that they call him Dad,
   and ah [....] but that was one of,   23
   those things,
   that ah in today's world you could even survive the trenches in France,
   with medication because everything is so much more,

   [....] LONG PAUSE
   the world is always producing new things,   24
   and so,
   [..] but then it is only for a short time,
   but the impact on us [...].

This instance also demonstrates that Tina's talk is not continuous enough to allow stanza segmentation. Tina responds to my questions regarding her children ("Ya, three/Mike, Didi, and Vicki and Jerry and Trevor and Elise") and where they are ("I: are they in LA?"/T: well ah ah well yes ... "). In Stanzas 21 and 22 she talks about her husband ("And N my husband and/ah his last name is Nichols"), and how her children call him "Dad" ("He he always goes by N/but the children ... call him Dad"). But soon after this, without warning, she jumps from talking about N to talking about how it "was one of those things that ah in today's world you could even survive the trenches in France...." On the face of it, these utterances in Stanza 23 seem completely incoherent; there does not appear to be any topical relationship between them and her previous utterances (about N and her children). Yet if we understand this stanza in terms of information she establishes elsewhere in our interaction ("My daddy died young/he died in the trenches in France.... they were filled with water ... and because of that he got tuberculosis ... "), it makes sense. Her talk about her children calling N "Dad" appears to have triggered off memories about her own father and she says:

> and ah [... .] but that was one of those things
> that ah in today's world you could even survive the
> trenches in France with medication because everything is so much more ...

The reason this segment comes across as egocentric is because she does not make clear to her audience the links between her previous utterances and her new information. The audience is thus left to establish the connections between Tina's idea about N's being called "Dad" and her own father not surviving the trenches.

Although one might be tempted to view the above utterances as new topic-initiating utterances, they are not really so because Tina has discussed her father some 30 utterances before. Coulthard (1977) called this *skip-connecting*. Chafe (1974) maintained that in such instances the speaker operates exclusively from a personal point of view by "extrapolating into the hearer's mind something that is really in his own mind" (p. 130). Such egocentric speech, according to Hutchinson and Jensen (1980), points to a reversal of a more primitive cognitive state, a prominent feature in their study of the language of the senile elderly.

THE EXTENT OF CONNECTED SPEECH IN HER DISCOURSE

Just as I parsed Tina's discourse at home and with N into segments of three connected ideas to get a sense of the degree of continuity in her speech, I also parsed her talk at the center. Of a total of 208 utterances, 131 can be grouped into segments of 3 lines. This yields 43.6 sets of connected lines. This means that 63% of her talk allows such segmentation compared with 93% in her talk at home. Table 4.1 lays out this contrast. I have included the percentage of talk that allows stanza segmentation in her interaction with her husband.

The difference in the extent of continuous speech in Tina's talk at home and at the center is, I believe, partly a result of extended dyadic pauses (classified as a discontinuity element on the continuity–discontinuity con-

TABLE 4.1
Percentage of Connected Speech in Tina's Talk in the Three Interactions

With Me at the Day-Care Center (%)	With Me at Home (%)	With N at Home (%)
63	93	2.25

tinuum discussed in chap. 2) evident in our latter interaction. These pauses, I believe, impede Tina from engaging in recall. However, before examining segments of our interaction that illustrate this, I briefly discuss extended pauses in general and some ways in which they can threaten interactions.

EXTENDED PAUSES AS DISCONTINUITY DEVICES

We are all familiar with times when interactions do not go smoothly, when we as interlocutors feel that miscommunication of some sort or another may have occurred. A number of studies have demonstrated that persons given to long pauses in conversation (long response latency following the completion of a previous turn by a partner) tend to be less socially skilled (McLaughlin & Cody, 1982). Biglan, Glaser, and Dow (1980) found that socially anxious women had more than 4-second silences in 5-minute conversations than socially non-anxious women. Wiemann (1977) treated 3-second pauses as *interaction management errors* and found that in combination with interruptions and unilateral topic switches, long latencies of response are related to lower ratings of communicative competence. Lapses/silences thus carry negative connotations of communicative failure.

As McLaughlin and Cody (1982) pointed out, most studies relating pauses to competency ratings have examined silences at the monadic level, in which interactional breakdown has been attributed to one participant. I feel, however, that silences can, in some cases, also be dyadic occurrences. If we understand conversation as a coordinated activity, one sustained through joint effort, then it would make sense to view lapses/silences as joint communicative failures, failures on the part of both (or all) participants. The following examples illustrate what I mean.

EXAMPLE 6
B: I get up about 5:20
A: Yeah
B: Go to workout at 5:45,
     work out-work out for an hour
     and 15 minutes in the morning and

>   then-except on Wednesdays—
>   on Saturdays we work for 3 hours
>   and every afternoon from 3:30 to 6:00
> A: Yeah
>   [3-second silence]
>   (McLaughlin & Cody, 1982, p. 300)
>
> EXAMPLE 7
> B: I think after a while they—their country's gonna==
> A: ( )
>   they're
> B: go under
> A: really
> B: You know, when it does it'll be—then it'll be complete chaos, and nobody'll be safe, especially Americans
> A: uhhuh
> B: So-oh
> A: Hmmm
>   (3.3-second silence)
> B: So that's my answer
>   (McLaughlin & Cody, 1982, p. 300)

McLaughlin and Cody pointed out that although A is the last speaker prior to the lapse in both examples and "B as a consequence is charged with a 3+-second response latency, the lapse is clearly due, in part, to A's consistent failure to provide anything more than minimal responses to B's utterances" (p. 301). The onus of sustaining the talk falls on B, because A opts to take passing turns (with "So-oh" or "really") rather than to advance the topic. However, it could be argued that B is also at fault for failing to recognize A's lack of interest in the topic. The lapses result on the part of both interactants. There is discontinuity between the utterances (in the preceding examples) inasmuch as one speaker has not gauged the other speaker's involvement. If continuity is a crucial feature in sustaining meaningful interaction, then extended pauses/delays can seriously threaten to derail the interaction (as they do in the preceding instances). Keeping in mind our concern here with narrative interactions, extended pauses (resulting from participants misgauging each other's intentions and involvement) could lead to discontinuity in the development of the emergent story. Certainly my interactions with Tina at the day-care center evidence this.

Extended Pauses in my Interactions With Tina at the Day-Care Center

Extended pauses in my interaction with Tina occur because both Tina and I are not assessing each other's cues accurately. These pauses, as the analyses point out, occur at transition-relevant places, points where one speaker has finished a turn and the other has not yet taken a turn. My operational definition of *prominent silences* is those silences that are 3 or more seconds long (indicated by three dots in square brackets [...]) that occur "subsequent to the recognizable completion of a turn constructional unit" (Sacks, Schegloff, & Jefferson, 1978), such as a sentence, independent clause, phrase, or lexical item. The opening segment of our talk in the day-care center illustrates this.

EXAMPLE 8
V: Tell me about yourself Tina

T: oh I have,   1
     I am one of three sisters and ah,
     ah no brothers unfortunately,
     and ah we always wanted brothers, [I: did you}
     and we didn't have any.
     —[...]
     ...

V: what's her name?
T: her name is Barbara Lee,   4
T: She's off.
     —[...]

V: is she older than you?
T: yes, uhuh,   5
     —[....]

V: do you have other sisters?
T: Barbara Lee is an ah is she,   6
     —[...]

We see several pauses in this segment alone. In each case pauses occur at potential transition-relevant places (TRP's) where I, as subsequent speaker, delay coming in. This delay is a deliberate strategy on my part intended to facilitate extended talk from Tina. As Mishler (1986) points out, when interlocutors remain silent "after the initial response, neither explicitly acknowledging or commenting on the answer nor proceeding immediately to the next question, respondents tend to hesitate, show signs of searching for something else to say, and usually continue with additional content" (p. 57). However, Tina has obviously not gauged my intention here, in that she has not understood that my silences are cues for her to keep talking. As far as she is concerned, she has answered my questions and is waiting for me to take my turn. The extended delay, then, disrupts the continuity of our interaction: Tina does not recognize the intention behind my delays, and I do not recognize Tina's expectations. This is evident in our exchange about her trip to India as well.

EXAMPLE 9
V: Is there any event that stands out in your memory about your stay there?
T: [says nothing] 30
—[...]

V: can you recall any event about India, Tina?
T: we stayed in the hills, 31
it was beautiful and fascinating.
—[...]

V: Tell me about one incident during your stay there
T: it was beautiful. 32
—[...]

We see Tina not responding at all to my prompt in Stanza 30, and after a significant pause (indicated by [...]), I prompt again: "Can you recall any event about India, Tina?" She responds this time, but only briefly ("We stayed in the hills/it was beautiful [...]") and does not develop this. We see another long pause at this turn at which I delay taking my turn. Evident in this instance, too, is the misalignment between my deliberate delay and Tina's conversational expectations. The same kind of misalignment seems to occur even after Tina has had an extended turn (i.e., after a narrative on her part). The following is an illustration.

EXAMPLE 10
T: well ah ah well yes, 21
Vicki and Jerry and Didi and N and I,
and N my husband and,
ah his last name is Nichols.

and ah ah he he always goes by Nick, 22
but the children don't go by Nick,
they call him Dad.
[..] and I like it that way [..],
I mean not had a father other than the father I lost in the war,
ah I like it that they call him Dad and ah.
—[... .]

but that was one of, 23
those things,
that ah in today's world you could even survive the trenches in France with,
medication because everything is so much more,

—[... .] LONG PAUSE
the world is always producing new things 24
and so
[..] but then it is only for a short time,
but the impact on us.
—[... ..] and ah [points to some children] aren't they cute? 25
V: ya

At the end of Stanza 22 and the beginning of Stanza 23 is a long silence. It is likely that the end of Stanza 22 marked the end of her turn. Tina waits for me to pick up my turn, and when I do not, she goes on talking. This occurs again at the end of Stanza 23.

In both cases, the misalignment does not seem to be because she has failed to interpret my delays as narrative cues—indeed, she continues talking even when I do not pick up my turn—but because Tina's conversational expectations are thwarted. The extended pauses occur at potential next-turns. She expects me to step into the interaction and take my turn, but I do not. Thus, our misgauging each other's turns interrupts the continuity of our interaction.

We see evidence of this in the following excerpt as well.

EXAMPLE 11
V: how old were you?
T: oh I was not a youngster at that   16
   particular
   point in time but he is always very busy,
   he works for Cal Tech,   17
   but we see a lot of each other too,
   we see to that I don't want a marriage where you are always away from your husband.
   it's not a good way to be at it,
   —[...]
   takes two for a marriage it does.   18

Tina is engaged in an extended turn in this instance as well: In Stanzas 16 and 17 she narrates about her husband and his busy schedule. At the end of that utterance we see a pause that signals the end of her turn, but, as in the earlier example, I once again do not take my turn, and Tina keeps talking.

These long pauses are discontinuous elements in that they hinder the smooth flow of talk. Our utterances seem, at several points, to be misaligned, with Tina not recognizing that delays on my part are signals for her to keep talking, and with my not recognizing that silences on her part are cues for me to step into the interaction. There do not appear to be as many pauses in our interactions at home. There are a total number of 83 turns in our interaction at the day-care center. Of these, 30 are dyadic pauses that are at least 3 seconds long. Likewise, the total number of turns in our interaction at home is 109, of which 12 are dyadic pauses.

The number of dyadic pauses in our interaction at the center was three times more than that of the pauses in our interaction at home, with pauses at the center constituting 36% of the turns and the pauses at home amounting to almost 11% (see Table 4.2). Setting thus appears to play a role in the relative (dis)continuity of her talk and our interactions.

TABLE 4.2
Dyadic Pauses in My Interaction With Tina at Home and at the Day-Care Center

Home (%)	Day-Care (%)
10.9	36

POSITIONING OF OTHER-REMINDING PROMPTS TOWARD THE END OF NARRATIVE SEQUENCES: A DISCONTINUITY ELEMENT

We now discuss some ways in which the positioning of (my) other-reminding prompts in ongoing interactions seem to inhibit recall from the patients and render the interaction discontinuous. The following exchange occurs soon after Amelia has finished narrating about her illness.

EXAMPLE 12
V: Uh well when you went to school tell me, what classes did you enjoy most? What did you like to learn about?
A: I like uh uhm, 1
  studying I liked ahm
  I think my best ... was uhm
  uh ... Melvin?
  Well, gosh
V: *did you like Math?*

A: that was my favorite 2
  [...]
V: that was your favorite
A: and uh ...
V: *well to be bookkeeper it had to be your favorite, right?*
A: well, but yes and it ah, 3
  that's true, it was,
  I liked it and I still do.

  I wish—I wish I could get things straight now but I can't, 4
  This last year has been uh, the hardest one.
V: I see
A: it's so hard to you know when you knew you were the one one,
  of the highest people in the class,
  That you couldn't even, can't um remember your own name hardly.

  And it's oh it's been awful, 5
  still getting used to it,
  I don't like it,
  I hate it.
V: I bet, it must be very difficult
A: But you have to do what you have to do the best that you can 6
V: *the last time I spoke with you, I still remember your positive attitude,*

	I'll never forget that.	
A:	Well you can still be nice to people and enjoy them,	7
	without uh I guess without knowing what their names are,	
	or what they do and that sort of thing,	
	but I would like it very much if I had my old self back.	
	[......]	
V:	how about any hobbies now?	8
	what do do you enjoy to do?	
A:	oh I go and work ah in ahm farming,	
V:	you like gardening, right	
A:	gardening, yeah.	

Lines 2 to 7 in the this segment indicate that Amelia is attempting to respond to my question regarding her favorite subject in school but without much success. In Line 8, I specifically prompt her with "Did you like Math?" to enable her to specify a subject, and we see her try to respond once again in lines 9 ("That was my favorite") and 11 ("and uhm ... "). Because I am aware that she had been a bookkeeper for most of her adult life, I remind her with "Well to be a bookkeeper, it had to be your favorite, right?" hoping that this will prompt her to say more. This time my reminding prompt is successful. We see Amelia engage in an extended turn wherein she provides some details about her current frustrations with her illness ("Its so hard ... when you can't remember your own name ... ") and recalls what it was like to be diagnosed with Alzheimer's disease (AD) ("This last year has been the ... hardest one ... I would like it very much if I had my old self back"). However, at the end of that segment there is a 6-second pause, after which I ask her about her current hobbies, which does not prompt any recall at all. In fact, we see her respond very briefly ("I go and work ah ahm farming ... gardening yeah").

One could come up with several interpretations of this. It is possible that Amelia is perceiving my utterance about her hobbies as too much of a topic change, because she has been talking about her illness immediately prior to my turn. However, given that we have been talking generally about what she enjoys doing, my utterance about her hobbies can be seen as topically related. Short-term memory loss is a common feature in AD (Swihart & Prizzolo, 1988), and it is possible that she has forgotten the general drift of the conversation. However, it is also possible that she interprets my utterance as pushing my agenda on her thoughts and therefore resists. Regardless what the topic was, however, or how each of us was construing it, it appears that my other-reminding prompts toward the end of narrative sequences tend systematically to derail the ongoing interaction and inhibit recall. The following segment from my interaction with Ed also illustrates similar derailing.

EXAMPLE 13
V: what kind of jobs did you have?
E: well, I was I was essentially a teacher all my life,
V: mm
E: I uh huh I was a teacher in high school in Chicago,   1
high school and uh I enjoyed that,
Then I went to college, University of Chicago.

and uh I was not married,   2
Uh-huh I finally found out I had a chance to go to England on a boat,
that had just come,
in in a freighter that had been unloaded.

And they I found out that,   3
they by curiosity (...),
I found out they had room for one passenger,
and uh and the fare was 90 dollars from Chicago to England.

and and as it turned out it was a a a it was uh unoccupied by this,   4
because it was saved,
saved for the captain's wife or one of the big investors in the company,
his wife or a couple of 'em could go.
but this trip it was not being used,   5
so I got her permission from my mother to go,
and I went,
and uh so (pause) we got to to (...) neck and neck race.

It was very slow,   6
We didn't get there on Tuesday,
We got there on Thursday,
and the Intrepid had won.

Well that wasn't very good,   7
but we got back to Chicago,
and un I sailed one way or another ever since.
V: I see
[....]

V: *did you do anything other than teaching?*
E: I ah uh you know I can't,   8
and ah I liked it,
V: liked teaching?
E: ah yeah ah but,
[...]

To my question about the kinds of jobs he did, Ed responds by saying he taught high school. After this, however, he launches into an extensive narrative (Lines 8 to 29) about his boat trip to England. At the end of Stanza 7 I remind him about his teaching career, a topic with which that segment had been initiated ("Did you do anything other than teaching?"), but we see that he does not launch into a narrative about it. In fact, the interaction falters at that point. It is possible that Ed perceives my question as too drastic a change in topic given what he had just been talking about. Possibly, he has forgotten that a question about his job had triggered his boat-trip narrative in the first place. It also is possible that he interprets my utterance as too much a pushing of my agenda and resists responding immediately.

There are an average of 2 other-reminding prompts out of an average of 8 narrative sequences that render the interaction discontinuous. This means that 25% of my (other-reminding) turns toward the end of narrative sequences threatened the interaction (see Table 4.3).

DRAWING IT ALL TOGETHER

In this chapter we examined some ways that Alzheimer interactions become discontinuous. We saw that Tina's narratives in the day-care center are relatively illformed in that they do not meet the wellformedness criteria quite as well as her talk at home does. Not only does she have difficulty taking extended turns but when she does, she needs extensive recipient scaffolding. We also see evidence of more egocentric speech, lapses of coherence, and sudden topic shifts in her talk at the center, all features characterized by Hutchinson and Jenson (1980) in their study of the senile elderly. The parsing of her speech into segments of three continuous ideas in both interactions reveals that she produces more connected speech at home than at the center.

We also saw that the illformedness of her talk was partially a result of misalignment in the interaction. All turns have to be understood in terms of prior turns in terms of the ways in (and sometimes even the extent to) which each interactant aligns his or her response in relation to the prior turn(s). In some cases continuity in the interaction is achieved, thereby facilitating meaningful interaction. In these cases, each participant meets the other participant's expectations by picking up the interactional cues, by contributing in a way that advances the topic meaningfully, and by demonstrating understanding of the prior turn(s). Although this was evident in our interaction at home (chap. 3), our interaction at the center evidenced several instances in

TABLE 4.3

Percentage of Self- and Other-Reminding Turns Toward the Beginning and End of Narrative Sequences That Lead to Recall

Other-Reminding Prompts Toward the End of Narrative Sequences (%)	Self-Reminding Prompts Toward the Beginning of Narrative Sequences (%)	Self-Reminding Prompts Toward the End of Narrative Sequences (%)
25	37	62.5

which Tina and I misgauge each other's conversational cues, resulting in extended pauses in our interaction. As the analyses in this chapter demonstrate, this was a result of Tina and me not assessing each other's conversational needs adequately. Tina, on occasion, does not realize that the reason I do not take my turn is because I want her to talk for an extended period of time. Likewise, I do not accurately gauge Tina's lack of involvement in the interaction. Our interactional cues are at cross-purposes, thus rendering our interaction relatively discontinuous. We noted too that there were fewer dyadic pauses in our interaction at home than at the center. These differences could be a result of several factors: Tina's relative discomfort at the day-care center, the various activities going on around her (there is a children's day-care center in the adjacent courtyard), and the frequent interruptions in our interaction (by her wandering attention).

We also saw how the positioning of other-reminding utterances toward the end of narrative segments contributed to threatening interactions. Given the findings in this chapter and those of chapter 3, this would mean that patients are more likely to recall if they are able to prompt themselves opposed to having the audience (me, in the present case) prompt them. On an average, 25% of my turns (toward the end of narrative sequences) fail to engage patients in recall, whereas 62.5% of self-reminding prompts (also toward the end of narrative sequences are likely to succeed.

CONCLUSION

These results, as well as those in chapters 2 and 3, call attention to the fact that interactions vary across contexts and, that narrative wellformedness partially results from the way that each participant gauges the different social phenomena. Often communication breakdowns occur because of cue misgauging between speaker and hearer, which in turn leads to participants stepping into interactions (me in the present case) at nonfacilitative moments. AD patients, like those of us who are normal, are sensitive to audience, setting, topic, time, and so forth. The influence of these different social features needs to be factored in when assessments are made about the patient's linguistic and communicative skills.

Consistent with the findings recorded in the previous chapter, some interactions facilitate better formed narratives from AD patients than others. A range of reasons for discontinuous interactions is possible, including participants (mentally) construing the several social factors differently—the previous utterance, the intention of the other interactants, the purpose of the activity the interactants are engaged in—and all at once. It is easy to see how interactions could get derailed and misgauging occur.

5

Repair as a Discontinuity Element: Examining Tina's Talk With N

> If we then ask about the nature and role of *psychological* genre—the reader's conception of what kind of story or text he is encountering or "recreating "—we are in fact asking not only a morphological question about the actual text, but also a question about the interpretive processes that are loosed by the text in the reader's mind.
>
> —*Jerome Bruner* (1986)

In the previous chapter we saw how Tina's ability to engage in recall is partially inhibited by dyadic pauses. We also saw how the particular positioning of my turns across the data inhibited recall. This chapter calls attention to another discontinuity element, namely repair, and another audience, namely Tina's husband, N. As we shall see, one reason why Tina's talk with N is illformed is because his extensive repair turns do not facilitate recall from her. In some cases they serve to alter her talk; in others they impede her ongoing turns. Before we get into the data, however, we begin by discussing the notion of repair and some ways in which I use this term in the analysis.

REPAIR AS A DISCONTINUITY ELEMENT

Repair utterances—the way Schegloff, Jefferson, and Sacks (1977) used the term—refer to those utterances made either by speaker or recipient toward altering/correcting a prior utterance. They call attention to two important distinctions in repair: first, self-initiated contrasted with other-initiated repair (i.e., repair by a speaker without prompting vs. repair after prompting) second, self-repair (that done by the speaker of the problem or repairable item), contrasted with other-repair (that done by another party). The following segments are illustrations of each:

Self-initiated self-repair
N: she was givin' me a:ll the people that were go:ne
this yea:r I mean this quarter y'//know ...
Other-initiated other-repair
A: lissena pigeons
B: quail, I think
Other-initiated self-repair
A: Have you tried a clinic?
B: What?
C: Have you tried a clinic?
(Schegloff, Jefferson, & Sacks, 1977, p. 364–368)

In my analysis, I focus exclusively on other-initiated repair turns that not only alter or correct the narrator's turn(s) but also obstruct the speaker from taking an extended turn. Given that Tina's husband had been informed about the larger aims of the study—namely to engage the teller in extended talk about him or herself—even recipient turns such as extensive collaborations or extensions that interrupt the narrator's ideas can get classified as repair utterances in that they interrupt the continuity of the ongoing story.

INABILITY TO PARSE TINA'S TALK WITH NICK INTO STANZAS

In chapter 3 we saw that Tina's talk with me lent itself to stanza parsing. Her talk with her husband, however, does not seem extended enough to allow this. The following excerpt illustrates what I mean.

EXAMPLE 1

N:	what else do you remember about your childhood Tina?	204
	you grew up in Preoria,	205
T:	ya	206
N:	and you mentioned your mother and ah [..],	207
	when you were a small girl there was some problem, at that time	208
T:	what was that N?	209
N:	well *you* tell me	210
T:	well my daddy died?	211
	well that was one,	212
N:	but before that	213
	[...]	
N:	you were ill/ very ill	214
	[...]	
N:	what did they do to you?	215
T:	Oh they cut a hole in my back they couldn't a give an anesthetic,	216
	because ah I was too far gone and ah	217

The previous excerpt, like the rest of her talk with her husband does not allow stanza parsing the way her talk with me does. This is partly because their interaction is in the form of a conversation.[1] Although the preceding segment—like her narrative to me in chapter 3—is about her childhood illness, it is much less informative. In this case, we learn about her illness, not from a storylike version, but from brief responses to prompts her husband has to make to draw the information from her. Tina appears to be unwilling to narrate when asked questions by him. When her husband, in the hope of getting her to talk, asks her about "what they did" to her when she was ill (Line 215), she does not go into the same detail she did when narrating to me. Instead, she replies in a direct but brief way that "they cut a hole" in her back, (Line 216) and that "they couldn't a give an anesthetic" because ... she was "too far gone" (Line 217).

We see this tendency elsewhere as well. In the following instance, Tina and N are talking about their stay in India and about her mother visiting them there.

EXAMPLE 2

N:	did your mother come over there?	20
T:	ya ya	21
N:	did she enjoy India?	22
T:	she wanted very much to go to India,	23
	I think she enjoyed it,	24
N:	what are some of things you began?	25
	remember the clinic? tell me about that.	26
T:	well the clinic was ah I worked there for a	
	while, right? [asks N]	27
N:	You helped set it up,	28
T:	ya, helped set it up.	29
N:	there was vacant block right? remember that?	
	across the street? [...]	30
	and you got two doctors,	31
T:	got two doctors/female and male,	32
N:	right and ah then?	33
	[...]	
	they would come over once a week and people would,	
	come from the villages would come in and,	34
N:	remember how you got it set up?	35
T:	got it set up,	36
	got it set.	

---

[1]This, however, is not to say that conversations cannot be parsed into stanzas. They can be. However, for stanzas to operate effectively, the conversation has to be co-constructed, with both parties contributing equally to the ongoing conversation. What happens in Tina's conversation with Nick is that Tina does not contribute enough to the interaction, causing an asymmetry in their interaction.

We can see in this example too that Tina's talk does not develop into a narrative. We see N asking her several questions: In Line 20, he asks Tina if her mother visited them in India, and as with the earlier example, Tina's response is again very brief. N continues prompting her ("Did she enjoy India"?, "What are some of the things you began?"/"there was a vacant block right? remember that?/remember how you got it set up?"), and for each question Tina's response is minimal. When, in Line 26, N says, "Remember the clinic/tell me about that," Tina's response demonstrates hesitation when she says, "I worked there for a while, right?" She is asking for clarification from N, implying uncertainty about that particular event. At no point in the this segment do we see her talk break into a narrative; it remains at the level of a conversation.

This tendency—of her talk not being connected enough to allow stanza parsing—is evident all through their interaction. In chapter 3, I parsed Tina's talk at home into segments of three connected ideas to get an idea of what percentage of her total discourse was continuous. I present a similar calculation of the connected speech in Tina's talk with Nick. Out of a total of 133 utterances, only 3 sets of 3 related lines are evident in Tina's talk. That is, only 2.25% of her talk with N was connected enough to allow 3-line parsing, figures that are in sharp contrast with her talk with me (see Table 5.1).

The fact that there is such a discrepancy in the amount of continuous speech Tina is able to produce with different interlocutors suggests that there is perhaps something in N's utterances that is impeding her narrative development. I would like to suggest that the illformedness in Tina's speech with Nick is partly due to his extensive use of repair utterances.

Examining N's Turns

One reason why Tina's talk to her husband remains at the level of conversation is because many of Nick's utterances are repair utterances that do not serve as continuers to further Tina's talk, but as interjections that impede/discontinue her extended turn. The italicized utterances in the following segments are such turns.

```
EXAMPLE 3
N:   how did he die?                                    236
T:   ah he had ah he had ah ah what was that            237
```

TABLE 5.1
Percentage of Connected Speech (at Least Three Connected Lines) in Tina's Talk With Nick and Me

With Nick (%)	With Me (%)
2.25	93

N:	he had gone to war?	238
T:	oh ya because he had gone into the	
	and service,	239
	ah he ah ah contracted tuberculosis,	240
N:	in the trenches	241
T:	in the trenches of France.	242
N:	and when he came back he still had it,	
	and ah	243
	penicillin had still not come in.	244
	[.] and what was really the sad thing, though Tina?	245
	when they put your dad in the hospital?	246
T:	oh we we ah [..] I don't know ah ah,	247
N:	you could only go into the you had to wave through	
	the window because you couldn't be near him	248
T:	no	249
	and ah he was such a loving person it was,	
	very difficult for him to be	
	isolated […].	250
N:	after that after he passed away	251
	you remember about that?	252
	his passing away?	253

EXAMPLE 4

N:	what are some of things you began?	25
	remember the clinic? tell me about that	26
T:	well the clinic was ah I worked there for a while,	
	right? [asks N]	27
N:	You helped set it up	28
T:	ya, helped set it up.	29
N:	there was vacant block right? remember that?	
	across the street? […]	30
	and you got two doctors	31
T:	got two doctors/ female and male,	32

EXAMPLE 5

N:	do you recall how you joined the Red Cross	
	right after college wasn't it?	59
T:	ya ya I was I ah I wanted to go,	60
	I always wanted to go and be part of the Red Cross,	61
	and so I I joined the Red Cross.	62
N:	you enjoyed it? you know they almost did not let	
	you join/	63
	remember Tina how hard it was to get in?	64
T:	Well ah I do,	65
	they thought ah ah they thought I ah I wouldn't,	
	ah ah [..] I think they thought I was just all for,	
	the uniform.	66
N:	no that might have been part of it,	67
	they were also concerned,	68
	that you'd gone to an all girl's school that you'd	
	been raised by your mother,	69
	and your two other sisters,	70

> *your father died when you were very*
> *very young,*   71
> *so you'd never lived with anybody but*
> *women,*   72
> *and you'd gone to school an all girl's*
> *school.*   73

We can see in these examples as well as throughout the Tina–N interaction that N's utterances are directed toward altering Tina's talk. As Nofsinger (1991) points out, "Participants routinely make various sorts of errors and then either revise what they have said or have the problems rectified by other participants" (p. 124). For instance, in Example 3, we see N repairing Tina's talk by introducing facts about her past that she has not yet thought to say. N's phrase "in the trenches" (Example 5, Line 241) is an extension of Tina's utterances about her father's tuberculosis. We see him altering her talk a few lines later as well. When Tina responds to N's question, "What was the sad thing … when they put your dad in the hospital?" (Line 246) with "Oh we we ah [..] I don't know ah ah…," N repairs her response to "You … had to wave through the window because you couldn't be near him" (Line 248).

Evident in both Examples 3 and 5 is that N's repair utterances sometimes take *extended turns*, turns longer than one would normally expect. In example 3, we see N extending Tina's talk about how her father contracted tuberculosis "in the trenches" (Line 241). Tina repeats this utterance in the next turn, and soon after, we see N engaged in an extensive turn from Lines 243 to 246 ("And when he came back he still had it and ah/penicillin had still not come in/ [.] and what was really the sad thing, though Tina?/when they put your dad in hospital?"). We see another extended turn on N's part in Example 5, where, from Lines 67 to 73, N repairs Tina's prior turn. In Line 66, Tina talks about why "they" gave her a hard time when she joined the Red Cross ("They thought I wouldn't/I think they thought I was just all for the uniform"). N repairs this by proffering his version ("They were also concerned that you'd gone to an all girl's school, that you'd been raised by your mother/and your two other sisters, your father died when you were very young/so you'd never lived with anybody but women and you'd gone to school an all girl's school").

Instances such as these highlight how N's repair utterances—whether brief or extended, collaborations or alterations—impede Tina's current turns, and thus contribute to the relative illformedness of Tina's talk.

N's Inability to Hear Tina's Narrative Cues

In the preceding sections we saw that N's repairing utterances contribute to their interaction remaining at the level of conversation. It can be argued, of course, that the reason Tina chooses to converse with her husband is because she does not feel the need to narrate to him because he has shared so much of her past and knows so much about it. Although this is a tempting argument, it does not account for instances when Tina talks about things that N does not share with her or does not know enough about. The following is an instance where they are talking about Tina's routine at the day-care center (something that N does not directly share, because he does not attend the center).[2]

EXAMPLE 6

N:	What's been happening at CAPS (the day-care center) lately?	1
T:	Oh not much, I uh we did we sort of did, [...]	2
N:	*what's happening with Francis? Is she still bothering you?*	3
T:	Ya she did, she took away my my ... she's horrible,	4
N:	*is she still taking away your stuff? She's always taking away your things,*	5
	I wonder if she took away your coat,	6
	remember you'd lost your coat at the center?	7
T:	ya and and ah she tore she tore my paper/ I ah I was,	8
N:	*What paper? were y'all drawing?*	9
T:	no no we we were using sticks (crayons?) and the paper ah was in,	10
N:	*What's her problem? I spoke to C (the manager of CAPS) about her and ...*	11

We see Tina beginning to narrate an event that occurred in the day-care center ("We sort of did [..]," Line 2), but not carrying on because N interrupts and asks her about Francis (Line 3). Then just as Tina is about to narrate concerning her recent spat with Francis ("She took away my my..."), Nick repairs her utterance with "Is she still taking away your stuff? ..."(Lines 5, 6, and 7). Tina tries yet again in Line 8 ("We were using sticks and the paper was in ..."), and once again, her effort is thwarted when N's repairing "What's her problem?" cuts in (Line 11).

Not only are N's utterances hindering Tina from narrating, but he also contextualizes every utterance of hers in previous knowledge he has of what happens in the day-care center. He is aware of previous tension between Tina and Francis and "overextends" this knowledge ("Is she still taking away

---

[2]This excerpt is taken from their conversation recorded 6 months after the previous recordings.

your stuff? She's always taking away your things," or "What's her problem? I spoke to the manager ... about her") to cover every utterance she makes. Even though all of us assimilate new information in the light of what we already know, N seems to do this to such an extent here that Tina does not get a chance to develop and communicate her new information. What I try to establish is that regardless of whether N has shared the event that Tina wants to talk about, he is not able to talk to her in a way that elicits a narrative. In other words, he is not able to "hear" her attempts at narrating.

Nick "Taking Over" in Other Interactions as Well

This inability on N's part to "hear" Tina's narrative attempts is not restricted to their interaction (Tina–N) alone. We see evidence of it in other kinds of interactions as well. In the following segment, the three of us are in a conversation, and once again we see N take over the floor.[3] In this excerpt we are talking about Tina's sewing skills. I had admired a quilt on her couch when we had the following conversation.

```
EXAMPLE 7
V:   It's professional Tina,                                    1
     you should have gone into business.                        2
T:   (laughs) Oh.. I made it a long time ago                    3
N:   She used to enter sewing competitions                      4
V:   Oh, tell me about it, Tina,                                5
N:   One time she sent one                                      6
     she didn't win I think                                     7
     and she wrote a letter complaining that.                   8
T:   ya and                                                     9
N:   and the winning things were very
     pedestrian,                                               10
     and she had made a sensational outfit.                    11
V:   hmmm                                                      12
T:   and I made,                                               13
N:   a skirt and a coat too, very stylish [..]                 14
     all out of silk and stuff,                                15
     so she wrote a letter protesting,
     [turns to her]                                            16
     what did the letter say when she
     wrote back?                                               17
T:   We was very sad that you was not happy,
     with ah our sewing machine contest (laughs).              18
V:   is that what the letter said?                             19
T:   [laughs]                                                  20
N:   ya the letter said "we was ..."                           21
```

---

[3] I recorded this conversation during one of my visits to their home.

T:	[laughs] ya you could tell she wasn't ah,	
	ah wasn't very educated.	22
V:	so you were quite a seamstress, huh Tina?	23
N:	*she was so into it,*	24
	she was always laying things out on	
	the floor.	25
T:	[laughs]	26
N:	*whenever I'd come home*	27
	on and there,	28
	I even helped with your hems, remember	
	that?	29
	I used to help you put pins?	30
T:	[laughs]	31
	[...]	

This segment, like the previous excerpts, displays N taking over Tina's turns. In this instance, too, as in the earlier one when they talk about her routine at the day-care center, we see N doing the talking for her. In Line 5, I specifically invite Tina to take the floor with "Tell me about it, Tina," but she does not get to tell me the story because N takes it on himself to tell it ("One time she sent one/she didn't win I think, and she wrote a letter complaining"). In Line 9, we see Tina trying to take a turn, but N does not hear her attempt and continues with the story ("a skirt and coat/very stylish"). In Line 17, N invites Tina to take the floor with "What did the letter say when she wrote back?" and after her response ("We was very sad that you was not happy with ah our sewing machine contest ...") N takes over the floor again. In Line 23, as in Line 5, I direct an utterance to Tina as a way of getting her to tell me the story ("So you were quite a seamstress, huh"), and once again, we see N responding instead of Tina ("She was so into it/she was always laying things out on the floor ...," Lines 24 to 30). It appears to be, then, that whether by themselves or in company, N is the dominant conversational participant in interactions that involve them both. This sense of his being in control is further highlighted in the following section in which his turns disallow Tina from engaging in extended talk.

Tina Unable to Establish Her Version of an Event

Another aspect about the Tina–N interaction is that although they have many shared experiences, N's extensive repair utterances hinder her from establishing her version of an event independently from N's. Tina lets N do the questioning and the prompting so that the final interpretation is more *his* than hers. Her responses to him are generally vague and brief. The following segment illustrates this. (N's utterances are italicized).

EXAMPLE 8

N:	do you recall how you joined the Red Cross	
	right after college wasn't it?	59
T:	ya ya I was I ah I wanted to go,	60
	I always wanted to go and be part of	
	the Red Cross.	61
	and so I I joined the Red Cross.	62
N:	you enjoyed it? you know they	
	almost did not let you join	63
	remember Tina how hard it was to get in?	64
T:	Well ah I do,	65
	they thought ah ah they thought I ah I wouldn't	
	ah ah [..] I think they thought I was just all for	
	the uniform.	66
N:	no that might have been part of it,	67
	they were also concerned,	68
	that you'd gone to an all girl's school, that	
	you'd been raised by your mother	69
	and your two other sisters,	70
	your father died when you were very very	
	young,	71
	so you'd never lived with anybody but	
	women,	72
	and you'd gone to school an all girl's	
	school.	73
T:	that's right	74

When N in Line 59 asks her, "Do you remember how you joined the Red Cross?" in the hope of getting her to narrate about it, Tina's response is a vague: "Ya ya, I always wanted to go ... " (Lines 60 to 62). We can see him doing much prompting: "You enjoyed it? you know they almost did not let you join/remember Tina? how hard it was to get in?" When she does come up with a tentative reason for their not letting her join ("I think they thought I was just all for the uniform," Line 66), N repairs her utterance by reminding her of the real reason: they thought she had only been around women and, thus, did not know much about men (Lines 67 to 73). Tina's response to this interpretation is "That's right" (Line 74). Tina appears to go along with N's version of an event. In fact, at no point do we see her even venturing to put forward her version of an event.[4] We see this demonstrated in the following segment as well.

---

[4]One could, of course, argue that the reason Nick does most of the interpreting is because he is aware that I am going to listen to the tape and so wants to clarify Tina's utterances for me. Although this is a plausible argument, I would like to stress that this is characteristic of the way Nick talks to Tina. There is plenty of evidence to demonstrate that even in interactions when I am present, Nick takes it on himself to do the interpreting or responding.

EXAMPLE 9

N:	*now seriously, Tina, how DID you meet me?*	101
T:	I didn't really,	102
	I just ahh I think some somebody told me about you,	103
	and ah so I decided ah my curiosity got the best of me and ah [..].	104
N:	*actually we both worked for a mutual friend who owned a restaurant [..].*	105
N:	*you know who that was?*	106
T:	sure sure that was was OUR restaurant,	107
N:	*well actually it was Jim Stockton's.*	108
T:	yeah Jim Stockton's	109
N:	*he owned a restaurant called the,*	110
T:	The Red Snapper	111
N:	*Smoke House.*	112
T:	what about the Red Snapper?	113
N:	*well Oh I think you are confusing it with another restaurant,*	114
T:	ohhh [...]	115
N:	*we both worked there,*	116
	I ah ah was going to graduate school at that time,	117
	it was a job worked at the restaurant at night, see,	118
	and you were working there also,	119
	so we got to talking and found out that we both played tennis.	120
	so you said to me once,	121
T:	[laughs]	
N:	*we'll go play tennis and I'll fix you brunch,*	122
	[...]	

As with the earlier segment, we see how N's repairs contribute to the sense of him "authoring" her story. When Tina responds to his question of the way they met ("I just ... think some somebody told me about you") in a way that he did not think was correct, he repairs her utterance to "Actually we both worked for a mutual friend who owned a restaurant [..]." We see him repairing her utterances in Lines 108, 110, and 112 as well, each time putting forward his interpretation. And finally from Lines 116 to 121 we see him engaged in an extended repair turn ("We both worked there/I ah ah was going to graduate school at that time/it was a job worked at the restaurant at night, see ...").

Nick Engaging Tina in Recognition Instead of Recall

Recipient turns, then, operate very differently in the two interactions: N's (repair) utterances do not seem to elicit narratives, whereas mine do. This brings us to the other issue that is a concern of this chapter: Why is it that, in Tina's interaction with N, it is N who takes the onus of reconstructing the events of Tina's past? Also, why is it that, in her interaction with me, Tina is able to manage the reconstruction by herself? Toward discussing these two issues, I would like to examine the nature of the prompts used by both interlocutors, because the prompts contribute, to a large extent, to the nature of the interaction. I would like to posit that the interlocutors engage Tina in different activities: N in recognition, I in recall. As established in chapter 2, context or setting is highlighted for recall, whereas the item or focal element is emphasized for recognition. We also established that recall manifested itself in narrative, with the patient being able both to sustain extended turns and to integrate audience turns into the ongoing story, whereas recognition disallowed either of these features. In the following analysis, I call attention to how N's prompts underscore item, thereby facilitating recognition, whereas my prompts emphasize context, thereby facilitating recall.

ANALYZING THE ROLE OF THE INTERLOCUTORS

Although both interlocutors talk to Tina about similar topics, the prompts they use are very different, influenced by the relationship each interlocutor shares with Tina and the shared knowledge between them. N's longstanding and intimate relationship with Tina makes him privy to aspects and events about her past that I, not knowing her well, do not have.

N's Event Specific Prompts

One aspect about N's prompts is that they are event-oriented: His questions and comments are specific and persistent in their attempt to get Tina to further develop what she says. In the following excerpt they talk about her illness.

EXAMPLE 10
N: *remember how old you were, then?* 218
T: Well I was three, four, five, 219
    I ran out in the rain [.]. 220
    it was so fascinating because it was,
    coming down you know, 221
    and ah I thought it was so beautiful, 222
    I got so enamored with it, 223
    so they they they [..] and they didn't,

	think they could pull me out of it but here I am.	224
	[laughs]	
N:	*but what did they do to you?*	225
T:	Oh they cut a hole in my back they couldn't a give an anesthetic,	226
	because ah I was too far gone and ah,	227
T:	ya, they had to they had to drain my lungs.	228
N:	*ya, so they put a tube in*	229
T:	ya [.],	230
N:	*and then they did,*	231
T:	ya	232
N:	*some other treatment something, like a lamp treatment.*	233
T:	ya	234
	they put me under the lamp you know,	235
	to ah ah	236
	what was that for, N?	237
N:	*for*	238
T:	just to drain,	239
N:	*to dry up*	240
T:	to dry me up.	241
	[…]	

In Line 218 we can see N trying to get Tina to narrate about her operation ("Remember how old you were then?"), and Tina gives the impression of complying when she goes into detail about how she ran out in the rain (Lines 219 to 224). But she does not go on, and N has to prompt her with "What did they do?" Once again Tina appears to try, but once again she does not sustain her effort ("Oh they cut a hole in my back they couldn't a give an anesthetic because ah I was too far gone and ah …," Line 226). We see this tendency in the following segment as well.

EXAMPLE 11

N:	*when did he die Tina?*	235
T:	ah he died quite early in fact he ah aha,	
	he was always such a friendly person you know,	236
N:	*how did he die?*	237
T:	ah he had ah he had ah ah what was that,	238
N:	*he had gone to war?*	239
T:	oh ya because he had gone into the service, and,	240
	ah he ah ah contracted tuberculosis,	241
N:	*in the trenches*	242
T:	in the trenches of France,	243
N:	*and when he came back he still had it and ah,*	244

	penicillin had still not come in,	245
	[.] and what was really the sad thing	
	though Tina?	246
	when they put your dad in the hospital?	247
T:	oh we we ah [..] I don't know ah ah,	248
N:	*you could only go into the you had to*	
	wave through the window because you couldn't	
	be near him.	249

As with the earlier example, we see that N's prompts and questions are event-specific: "When did he die?" "How did he die?" "Had he gone to war?" "What was the sad thing ... when they put your dad in the hospital?" Coupland, Coupland and Giles' term (1991), *overaccomodation*, can be effectively applied here. Coupland et al. use this term specifically to refer to miscommunication, in which one party appears to "go beyond" the necessary sociolinguistic style judged necessary on a particular occasion. Examples they provide are talking too loudly or being overly cautious. Although there does not appear to be miscommunication between Tina and N, I believe this term can be applied to segments such as the preceding. N's prompts can be seen as "overaccomodative" inasmuch as they appear to be overly persistent. Their event-specific, probing nature suggests that N feels responsible to pursue his effort at getting her to talk. If the interviewer were to remain silent "neither explicitly acknowledging or commenting on the answer nor proceeding immediately to a next question, respondents tend to hesitate, show signs of searching for something else to say, and usually continue with additional content" (Mishler, 1986a, p. 57). But we do not see evidence of pauses between turns in the Tina–N interaction. N is very much the active recipient (Mandelbaum 1989).

I am, on the other hand, a relatively passive recipient in Tina's interaction with me. In the following segment, for instance, except for the initial preface sequence (Sacks, 1974), which is almost always interactional, I do not participate at all.

EXAMPLE 12
V:	*how old were you?*	
T:	oh lets see,	
	I was in Kindergarten.	
V:	*ya, you were really young*	
T:	uhhuh	
T:	and ah I,	1
	daddy used to have to carry me,	
	and ah [...] you know,	
	it was a bad situation,	
	but it brought us all close together.	

and ah you see, they cut this wound on my back without anesthetic, [.] and I was just a teenager.	2
and ah it was ah, my mother didn't know they were going to operate on me and ah, I kept deteriorating and deteriorating and on. and I guess they felt they had to do something.	3
and I guess my mother was furious when she found out, that they had cut this hole in my back. and ah [… .], it was a painful situation.	4

Mandelbaum (1989) maintains that even a teller's extended turn is an interactive accomplishment of recipient and teller working together. Implicit in the recipient's nonparticipation is the "go ahead" signal for the teller to keep talking.

N Deciding What Tina Should Talk About

Another aspect of N's prompts is that they reveal N controlling what it is Tina should talk about. Because he knows the details of all the events, he does all the questioning, and he provides her feedback to further their interaction. This is evident in Example 13, which I have reprinted.

EXAMPLE 13
N:	what else do you remember about your childhood Tina?	204
	you grew up in Preoria	205
T:	ya [.]	206
N:	and you mentioned your mother and ah, […] when you were a small girl there was some problem at that time	207 208
T:	what was that N?	209
N:	well YOU tell me	210
T:	well my daddy died?	211
	well that was one,	212
N:	but before that […]	213
N:	you were ill very ill […]	214
N:	what did they do to you?	215
T:	Oh they cut a hole in my back they couldn't	

a give an anesthetic, 216
because ah I was too far gone and ah. 217

In Lines 204 and 205 we once again see N trying to get Tina to narrate about the illness she suffered in her childhood ("What else do you remember about your childhood Tina? you grew up in Preoria" and "There was some problem at the time, right?"). However, Tina is not able to place immediately what "problem" N refers to, and she says "What is that N?" (Line 209). In Line 211 she tries to guess what N is getting at with "My daddy died," but this is not the right answer. A little later, we see N providing more direct prompts: "You were ill for a while, right?" and then, "What did they do to you?" Tina finally realizes in Line 216 the specific event that N wants her to talk about and says "Oh they cut a hole in my back."

Another segment that evidences this tendency is the following.

EXAMPLE 14
N: *and when you'd got it in Red Cross*
what did they say to you, you
remember that? 75
T: they said I was ah ah ah they were
concerned, 76
that I would I would not be able to cope,
ah cope with it and ah ah they ah they ah, 77
I didn't know very much, 78
about men and ah. 79
N: *what did you say? how did you get in*
then? 80
T: Well I said no I, 81
I I said I definitely wanted to be in
the Red Cross, 82
so they said well they would ah
try me out 83
N: *well they contacted one of your former ah*
teachers, I think in college? 84

In this segment too, we see Nick controlling what Tina should say. In Lines 75 and 80 he asks her how she managed to get accepted by the Red Cross, and as in the earlier example, we see Tina trying to guess the response N wants her to make. But unlike the previous segment we do not see her make the correct guess, and finally we see N prompt her toward what he thinks is the correct response in Line 84 (that she got in because the Red Cross got in touch with one of her teachers in college).

N's prompts, in the preceding segments, are directed toward getting Tina to make specific responses, responses that he thinks are the right responses. We also see that he decides what she should talk about. He thus provides her specific prompts in rapid succession that encourage her to guess the event in question. We do not find this to be the case in her narratives to me. Because I do not know the events of her past, my questions are, compared to N's, vague and general ("When you look back on your childhood, Tina, what is it that stands out most?" or "Tell me about your marriage/what was that like?"). The open-ended nature of my questions places the onus of recalling squarely on Tina.

The peculiar nature of N's prompts call attention to an important point: Although they may be intended to make Tina *recall* certain events, they really serve only to make her *recognize* them. We saw in chapter 2 that the process of recall involves the process of *retrieving* and *deciding*, while recognition involves only the latter. An aspect about N's prompts (evident in its event-specific nature, as well as in the fact that he controls Tina's talk) is that he, by and large, does both the retrieving and deciding for her. Illustrations of N's highlighting the focal elements of her past for her are evident in certain prompts: "When you were a small girl there was some problem at that time, right?" or "what did they do to you?" or "What did you say?, How did you get in then?" In other words, he is the one engaged in recalling here. He constructs the scaffolding of Tina's past. Tina's role in their interaction seems to be limited to filling in the gaps of this scaffolding (which, as we have seen, she is able to do only occasionally). By taking on the onus of scaffolding her past, *N has become the repository of her memories*.

DRAWING IT ALL TOGETHER

The preceding analyses call attention to yet another way in which recipient turns can impede narrative development. Tina's talk with Nick is in sharp contrast to her talk with me in that the latter evidences much more connected speech (93%), speech that allows stanza segmentation. Her talk with N, however, remains at the level of conversations (with only 2.25% of connected speech), without meaningful development of stanzas. We also see that regardless of the kind of event that Tina and N talk about, whether it is something they have shared or something that N does not know much about (such as what happens at the day-care center, their interaction does not encourage her to narrate.

We can see that much of Tina's ability to narrate is tied to the recipient's behavior: in the way in which each recipient listened or interrupted, in the extent and nature of repairs that each recipient made, in the prompts that each recipient made to further talk (event-specific vs. open-ended), and in the feedback that each interlocutor provided toward sustaining the interaction. I am proposing, of course, that Tina might have been able to produce extended and meaningful talk with N as she did with me had the former interaction been facilitative. Had N's contributions to their interaction been such that they encouraged *recall,* an activity in which the narrator both retrieves and decides which event he or she wants to talk about, then in all likelihood N would have been able to elicit narratives from Tina. But because N does both the retrieving and the deciding, all that is left for Tina is to recognize the event.

Because N bears the onus of recall in their interaction, the interpretation of events they talk about seems to be more his than hers. As we saw in Section 3, the event-specific nature of his prompts channels their talk in particular directions, toward interpretations that N thinks are correct. Although it is possible that Tina may view the event in question in the same way as N, the point I wish to underscore here is that she is not being given a chance to establish *her* version of the event. At no point in their interaction are we able to see Tina even *trying* to negotiate with N about another interpretation of a shared event. At points when Tina does try to narrate (when the onus of deciding and retrieving the event in question could be entirely hers), N's extensive repair utterances hinder him from hearing her narrative cues.

Yet, can N be faulted for not being able to hear Tina's cues? Confronting his wife's growing inability to recall her (and their joined) past on a daily basis contributes, no doubt, to his overcompensation for her, manifesting itself in his tendency to overrepair her utterances. It is quite possible that this is the only way he knows of how to preserve her past and her face for her, because she is losing the ability to maintain them for herself.

6

A Schematic Understanding of Repetition in an AD Life Story

> Frequently and with deliberation and respect we should revisit our early memories—memories which do not fade and which hold the incorruptible essence of emotion. These memories are the parts of us which change least with time, perhaps because they come from periods when we were most in tune with time; and coming back to them we come upon ourselves—not the harried, hustling, temporary selves we see when we compromise with the mirror, but rather what Yeats called "the pilgrim soul," at once most our own and most confluent with the race.
>
> —*Robert Grudin* (1982)

This chapter shifts focus somewhat, in that it concentrates primarily on an Alzheimer's disease (AD) patient's self-narratives across time. I attempt to present a more holistic picture of this patient than I did of Tina, by combining ethnographic details of the patient's social world with a microanalysis of her narratives. I do so primarily because much happens in the patient's social world that, I believe, at least indirectly exacerbates her already deteriorating condition and makes her hold on the world and language that much more tenuous. The analysis of her social world includes in-depth descriptions of the day-care center and her life there, as well as a review of her major life events up until the time I started working with her.[1] The analysis of her discourse entails a schematic analysis of repetition in her talk toward understanding ways in which her overall interpretive schema remains the same despite the ravages of the disease and a nonfacilitative social environment.

---

[1] I was able to put together parts of Ellie's life on the basis of what people who knew her well told me about her. These included her daughter, caretaker, manager of the day-care center, and a friend from the apartment complex she used to live in.

Tracing her progressively deteriorating condition across the span of a year and a half, I argue that what can be regarded as "incoherent" and illformed speech in latter stages of the disease may be seen to make sense if understood in context of the patient's previous recordings when her linguistic skills were not quite as impaired.

BACKGROUND

A tenet central to cognitive psychology is understanding how information is encoded and processed in the brain. Several cognitivists maintained that we encode and store all information in the form of *schemata* (or "gists" or "categories," depending on the theory embraced) and that these schemata serve as organizational structures by which we process current and past information. Rumelhart (1980) maintains that schemata play a central role in the comprehension of verbal information. Schank and Abelson (1977), focused on the storage of information and used the term "scripts" to explain information encoding. Using schema theory to explain aspects of human behavior, cognitive anthropologists such as D'Andrade (1992) viewed schemas as cognitive structures within which cultural motivations and goals are embedded.

The analysis in this chapter follows similar lines inasmuch as it attempts a partial understanding of how (autobiographical) information has gotten encoded and bound in the repeated segments of talk so prominent in the discourse of AD patients. Previous psycholinguistic research on AD discourse has documented repetition (referred to as *echolalia* in the literature) as a feature that contributes to incoherence in AD speech and has understood it largely in terms of the progressively deteriorating nature of the disease (Hunt, 1990; Kempler, 1991; Ulatoska et al., 1988). This chapter, in contrast, examines such segments of talk in an attempt to understand, not how they contribute to the semantic emptiness in AD discourse, but how they reflect cognitive representations of particular autobiographical events. Such an analysis should help us view these segments as illustrative of the AD patient's *remnant*, meaning-based discourse skills (Ellis, Duran & Kelly 1994; Villaume, Jackson & Schouten 1989), in which the focus is on language wellness as opposed to language deterioration.

Toward this end, I do a detailed schematic analysis of the events in the life stories of Ellie, an AD patient recorded twice over a period of a year and a half. Previous schematic analysis of normal life stories (Strauss, 1992) has argued that bound segments, because of their self-contained nature, get only weakly linked to the rest of the teller's knowledge structure. However, I argue that bound segments, self-contained as they are, have strong links with the other unbound event schemata in the speaker's story, that meaning-based connections can be established between the bound and unbound event schemata as well as between the event schemata and the teller's larger interpretive framework. (I discuss the criteria for establishing boundedness in the section that discusses establishing bound talk in AD speech.) I also point out ways in which Ellie's interpretive schema is evident a year and a half later when her condition has deteriorated considerably and her discourse strategies have become more text-based and impaired (Ellis et al., 1994; Villaume et al., 1989). (Meaning-based and text-based narrative-discourse are discussed presently).

ELLIE'S SOCIAL ENVIRONMENT: ABOUT THE DAYCARE CENTER

Located in a poorer, run-down, and seedy part of town, the day-care center Ellie attends is in a neighborhood that has a reputation for drug trafficking and prostitution. The street on which the center is located is, on the whole, quiet but dirty. There is litter on the streets, and people passing by (both elderlies and others in the neighborhood) do not hesitate to litter it more. Most of the vehicles on this street are vans: vans that transport elderlies from their homes to the center, vans with hot meals (meals on wheels) for the elderly citizens, and vans selling fast food. The number of older citizens around the building—some sunning on benches outside, others slowly shuffling over the steps of the center, still others being taken on walks with aides—easily identifies this place as a center for the aged.

The elderlies attending this center are ethnically diverse—Whites, Blacks, Hispanics, Asians—and they cover a full range of the aging cycle from "young-elderlies" who are still relatively agile and energetic to "old-elderlies" who are wheeled in or who need help walking. The inside of the center seems modern with automatic doors that swing open just as you are about to step in. Immediately to the left is a receptionist sitting at a desk on which is a televised camera that screens goings on in other parts of the center. This entrance leads into a large sunny room with a fiberglass sky roof, the walls of which are devoted either to bulletin boards (about a variety of things including upcoming trips, rental homes, van services, special classes for the elderly, prayer meetings, etc.) or benches. Rarely are these benches empty. Many of the normal elderlies seem to love to spend their time here knitting, chatting, cutting up grocery coupons, and exchanging news about children, family members, health, love affairs, prices, and homes. Clearly this space is an area of heightened sociability.

Toward one end of this room is a large enclosed space where the AD patients (about 12 to 14) are supervised. Except for people who work in this room—aides, social workers, family members, administrators and occasional volunteers such as—everybody else stays out. Patients are not allowed to leave this room except to go to the restroom, in which case they are always accompanied by one of the aides. The door of the room is always closed from the inside, leaving the impression that the outside world has collapsed to the size and perimeters of this one room, a room and world inhabited by other elderlies in different stages of the same ailment. One wonders whether this kind of isolation within the center itself does not strongly reinforce the social isolation that patients must have begun to feel with the onset of aging and the AD.

There is isolation of yet another kind, namely in the patient–staff interaction. In fact, "interaction" is a misnomer in that it implies bidirectional communication. Communication between patient and aide at this center is at best unidirectional, extending only from the aide to the patient. Patients are seldom asked what he or she would like to do, say, draw or sing. They either have to do what the aides want them to do or allow the aides to do to them what they want to do. What gets done to and for the patient depends partially on the classification to which the aides have assigned him or her. There are those who are "good" because, on the whole, they can manage their baths, meals, and general moving around. These are generally patients who are in the mild to moderate stages of AD, who occasionally experience forgetfulness (e.g., they may forget how to get back to the room from the restroom, which is why everyone is accompanied back and forth). Then there are the "chair" types who are encouraged not to leave their chairs. They are the patients that need to be taken to the restroom every few hours because they forget to ask. They are also the ones that need to have their meals brought to them. Finally, there are the "do-nothing" types (those in the severe stages of the disease) who do not seem to be able to manage anything. They cannot comprehend what is said to them, so they do not seem to participate in anything: They do not talk, they do not eat until they are fed, they do not even voice the need to go the restroom. Everything has to be anticipated by the aides: their thoughts, needs, wishes, discomforts. In this last type are the ones that seem to live in a vacuum: They appear to have lost their hold on language—the key to the outside world—and to themselves.

Life in this room is highly routinized. The day officially starts at 10 a.m. with simple exercises that everybody performs to music, after which everybody sits in small groups at tables to paint, draw, or solve jigsaw puzzles. Occasionally, these patients are encouraged and taught to make things such as bracelets, masks, or figurines out of plastic, string, plastecine, or paper.

The finished articles are then hung up for display or put in a glass case that stands at one corner of the room. Activities such as these go on until 11:30 a.m. at which point lunch, catered by a "meals on wheels," is brought in. The lunch typically consists of a quarter pint of milk, some meat, vegetables, and a roll of bread, all of which taste extremely bland. After lunch, the patients often engage in a game. Sometimes they are made to form a large circle and toss a ball between them with sponge-covered bats. At other times, they are encouraged to dance to music. This goes on until 4 o'clock in the afternoon, after which these patients are picked up by their family members or driven back to their homes.

LOCATING ELLIE IN THIS CONTEXT

When I began work at this center, Ellie was classified a good type. She came across as someone who was quietly independent, not talking very much and generally amenable to whatever the aides wanted her to do. In fact, she was one of their favorites because she did not make demands or seek special attention.

Ellie was born in Milwaukee but was raised in Chicago where she spent a rather unhappy and unstable childhood. Her parents divorced when she was 3 years old, and this is something from which Ellie has never fully recovered. Her father, whom she adored, married again, and Ellie found her stepmother hostile. She ran away when she was about 14 and got a job as a help in a Jewish family. She was quite happy with this arrangement because the family that took her in lived near her father, and she was able to see him occasionally.

Ellie had three or four long relationships with men and several shorter ones on the side. She was married twice, both times to air force pilots. Both marriages were financially secure but unhappy, because both husbands "chased after other women." She had a daughter by her second marriage, but she and her daughter are not, and never have, been close. When her daughter was about 14 years old she was arrested for prostitution, taken out of Ellie's charge, and put into a foster home.

For most of her life, Ellie worked as a waitress at bars in big hotels where she met most of the other men in her life. Others I talked to regarding Ellie said she drew men to her like flies, both in her younger days and at the day-care center. In fact, most of the men in the center know her well and flirtatiously hail her as "boom boom Ellie" because of her "oomph," Even today, one can see the remnants of a beauty: startling green eyes and graying red hair.

Ellie did not really keep in touch with her family except for a sister that lived in California where she acted in small movie roles. About 10 or 12 years ago, her sister fell dreadfully ill, and Ellie traveled to California from Chicago to take care of her. Her sister died a couple of days after Ellie arrived, and Ellie inherited all her money and possessions. At this point, Ellie, decided to give up her job as a waitress in Chicago and move to California. She found herself an apartment in a complex where many other elderly lived. Ellie was at this time in her mid-60s, and it was around then that Ellie was diagnosed with Alzheimer's disease. Two of her friends (whom I interviewed to find out more about Ellie) took her to the Los Angeles County Hospital where she underwent a series of tests including the Boston Naming Test and minimental tests. The results indicated features commonly associated with dementia—short-term memory loss, trouble with finding words, frequent repetition, problems with concepts—and she was diagnosed to be in the mild to moderate stages of the disease. Her friends also got her to join the day-care center that she has been attending ever since.

Small things started to go wrong with Ellie around this time. She used to frequent a neighborhood bar where she would pick up men and bring them home. Being alone, vulnerable, forgetful, and generous, Ellie was soon relieved of a lot of her money. She got involved with an alchoholic named Tom, and her relationship with him lasted about 3 years. Tom used to live in the same apartment complex, so it was easy for him to financially abuse her, which he did. The other elderly folk in the building who had "old fashioned ideas about aging and sex", did not approve of Ellie having Tom in her bed and one morning marched into her apartment and bodily evicted him and his things. It was soon after her breakup with Tom that I recorded her for the first time.

A notable feature in Ellie's talk at this time was the way she repeated chunks of information. As mentioned at the outset, these chunks represent frozen ways in which she has encoded specific bits of autobiographical information and made sense of her past. Before we get into analyzing them, it might be useful if I review previous research on information storage and some psycholinguistic perspectives on repetition.

SCHEMATA, INFORMATION STORAGE, AND AUTOBIOGRAPHICAL ENCODING

As mentioned at the outset of this chapter, several cognitive psychologists believe that all humans store information in the form of *schemas*, conceptual structures by which our brains absorb, categorize, retain, and identify information. The encoding of an event in our minds implies the encoding of a series of frames—that includes both verbal and nonverbal representations, which captures both action and persons involved in it.[2] Not only do we process most of our new information in light of previously stored schemata, but we also interpret new information in the light of the existing schema. That is, if aspects of the new information being received is congruent with an existing schema, then it is likely that this schema will be activated when interpreting that event. However, there may be times when the information received cannot fit with existing schemata. In such instances, the new information could be incorporated as an exception, or correction. For instance, if information about a person's behavior at a restaurant includes the fact that the person pulled out a gun, then "pulled out a gun" would be regarded as a correction that qualifies the encoding of the information as simply "eating at a restaurant." This kind of information is more likely to be retained because of its unusual nature because it stands out from other more typical frames involved in an "eating at the restaurant" schema (Wyer & Srull, 1984). Extending this reasoning to autobiographical memories, would mean that the most vivid memories about ourselves are frames that stand out or are at least different from the innumerable others that make up the events of our lives. Because schemata are encoded in terms of their social contexts, the cognitions associated with the act of encoding them may often be important components that trigger retrieval. This is particularly true of autobiographical memories in that certain contexts (topics, utterances, people, settings) may trigger the retrieval of certain memories.

Wyer and Srull (1984) proposed that units of information can get chunked over time on the basis of certain connections (temporal, chronological, emotional). These links demonstrate ways in which a person has made sense of event sequences, of the ways in which he or she connects pieces of information. With repeated tellings, these chunks of information can get bound. All of us have, at one point or another, conjoined event sequences while narrating, either about ourselves, other people, things, or events. When rehearsed over time, the associations that we make between these event schemas get set, and the information sequence gets bound and closed. (I illustrate this point with AD data in a later section which discusses criteria for establishing bound talk in AD speech.) Abelson's (1965) definition of bound storage sums this up effectively: He refers to these self contained cognitive units as

> "opinion molecules" ... [which] give you something to say and think when the topic comes up.... These sorts of opinions are often quite impervious to other levels of

---

[2] Abelson (1968) drew an analogy between the frames of a script and a comic strip, in which each may have both a caption denoting the event and a picture containing many details about the people, objects, and events involved. "These may include characteristics of oneself as participant or observer in the situation, such as one's behavior or even one's subjective reactions or thoughts that occur while the events take place" (Wyer & Gordon, 1984, p. 96).

argumentation, because of their complete, closed, molecular character. It is as if the opinion-holder were saying, "what else could there possibly be to add?" (p. 27)

Strauss (1992) argued that the self-contained nature of such units keeps them from being integrated into a larger structure. However, a later section detailing explanatory statements and organization of event schema demonstrates how these closed units get integrated into larger interpretive schemas to produce relatively meaning-based narrative texts.

ABNORMAL REPETITION: SOME PSYCHOLINGUISTIC PERSPECTIVES

Referred to as *echolalia* in the literature, abnormal repetition comes under the broad rubric of *perseveration*, which indicates the "persistent repetition or continuation of an activity once started" (Buckingham, Whitaker, & Whitaker, 1976, p. 329).[3] Being disordered in nature, Buckingham et al. posited that perseveration is accentuated under conditions of weakness, inattention or out of frustration to do a particular task. Distress-causing conditions, too, have been known to generate perseveration (Goldstein, 1948).[4]

Linguistic perseveration or echolalia refers to the repetition of linguistic features/utterances in a disordered fashion. Buckingham et al. found that perseveration frequently occurs on tasks such as repetition and naming aloud. For instance, JT, when asked to repeat "window," said "red window." Next, when asked to repeat "banana," she said "a back window" (p. 334). The perseverate in the first instance was repeated as the correct response to the second stimulus item. A similar tendency was found in the naming tasks. The following is an illustration:

STIMULUS	RESPONSE
hand	patient could not name it
car	/hæ / / hæ / uh….
girl	that's a /hæ /uh… .

(Buckingham et al., 1979, p. 335)

---

[3]For studies on "normal" repetition see Bennett-Kastor (1978), Johnstone (1987), Keenan (1977), Ochs (1979), Tannen (1989).

[4]The presence of perseveration had been documented in specific language-impairing diseases. Eisensen (1971, 1973) discussed perseveration in aphasics and said it could signal a behavioral breakdown. He also stated that "perseveration, in general, may be the human mechanism's way of reacting to situations which demand adaptations and call for responses which the individual is not capable, momentarily or chronically, of making" (1971, p. 1258). He also pointed out that nonbrain-damaged persons may perseverate when fatigued or when required to perform a task more rapidly or with more frequent changes.

The word "hand," which the subject attempts to articulate (but does not succeed in doing) is later perseverated in other naming tasks. Linguistic perseveration also can also be seen in spontaneous talk. Buckingham et al. (1979) provided the following as an illustration:

> uh, I can't even say it ... isn't that funny ... /dri??, uh ... used to ... isn't that funny, I can't /dri?/ I used to.... (p. 336)

Here the speaker attempts to find certain words and, when she is not able to do so, begins to perseverate those words she *is* able to produce. The phrases "I can't," "Isn't that funny," and "used to" are all repeated twice in two lines, contibuting to the talk being disjointed and out of context.

Research done on the language of patients with autism (Rutter, 1966) and dementia (Ulatowska et al., 1988) also reveals the presence of verbal perseveration. Freeman and Gathercole (1966), in their study of schizophrenic and dementia patients, documented several different patterns in perseveration. They found that dementia subjects were most likely to evidence *ideational perseveration* (the repetition of an idea after an intervening response) and *impairment of switching* (repetition of an idea after an intervening stimulus). The study on dementia discourse by Bayles, Tomoeda, and Kasniak, (1985) also documented repetition of ideas after an intervening response.

Although the present chapter focuses on repetition in Alzheimer discourse, it does not call attention to the functions of repetition (the way much research in discourse analysis has done). Neither does it aim to observe the kinds of repetition evident in dementia discourse (the way psycholinguistic research has done). Instead, it attempts to explore the ways in which segments of repeated AD talk reflect the remnant meaning-based discourse skills that the patients have retained.

MEANING-BASED VERSUS TEXT-BASED (NARRATIVE) DISCOURSE

Meaning-based and text-based discourse strategies—terms generally associated with interactional involvement (Cegala, 1981; Ellis et al., 1994; Villaume et al., 1989)—capture degrees of speaker involvement in conversations. "Meaning-based strategies require a participant to attend to deeper, more elaborate meanings ... " (Ellis et al., 1994, p. 148), thus, requiring, a relatively high degree of cognitive involvement on the part of the speaker. Text-based strategies, in contrast, are indicators of relatively low involvement in which the participant orients "only to surface textual information from the most recent utterances and does not integrate this into a larger and more complex mental representation...." (Ellis et al., 1994, p. 148). Although these terms are generally used to capture interactional features, for the purposes of this study, I borrow them toward the analysis of narratives/life stories. Because the present study concentrates solely on patient turns (and not on interactional features), "meaning-based" discourse is understood in terms of the patient's ability to engage in extended and meaningful narratives with explanatory statements (discussed in detail in a later section analyzing Ellie's life history), whereas "text-based" discourse refers to the patient's inability to cognitively engage in such talk. (As will be shown later, explanatory statements render Ellie's talk as meaning-based by linking her life events to her overall interpretive schema.)

Rather than regard meaning-based and text-based strategies as dichotomous terms, I suggest that we view them as different points on a continuum. (For more information on different kinds of discourse continua, see Chafe, 1982; Tannen, 1982; Ramanathan-Abbott, 1993). What is relevant in discussing any use of language is placing it within both a discourse continuum and larger sociocognitive arena of which the continuum is a part, not identifying it only as meaning-based or text-based. All of us as speakers, for a variety of reasons, range across a certain portion of this continuum, being more cognitively involved and meaning-based in certain contexts and particular times than others. We see from the analysis of Ellie's life stories, that there is a variation in her discourse abilities across time: Her talk is relatively more meaning-based in the first recording, more text-based in the second.

CRITERIA FOR ESTABLISHING BOUND TALK IN AD SPEECH

Before we go into examining the bound nature of some segments in AD talk, I must establish what *boundedness* means and the criteria I apply to judge it. I take Roger Abelson's (1968) definition of bound storage (discussed in an earlier section) as the operational definition for this study. These self-contained "opinion molecules" are bound in that they strongly demarcate the boundaries within which they are held. I discussed earlier how sets of autobiographical events get unitized on the basis of certain connections (temporal, chronological, and emotional), and the ways in which they become closed chunks of information with repeated tellings. Implied in the bound nature of these chunks are the cognitive links (Strauss, 1992) or connections that the teller has established between the ideas that

EXAMPLE 1
a. my father remarries and my stepmother
   took one look at me,
   and she could kill me.
   (Ellie, day-care)
b. so he got remarried and she took one look
   at me and hated the sight of me.
   (Ellie, day-care)
c. so he had remarried,
   my stepmother took one look at me and felt
   like she'll kill me right away.
   (Ellie, day-care)

EXAMPLE 2
a. my daddy had tuberculosis
   all his life,
   he got it in the trenches of France.
   (Tina, at home)
b. my daddy died very young,
   he died in the trences of France,
   dreadful place.
   (Tina, day-care)

EXAMPLE 3
a. I met my wife in East LA,
   I met her at a dance.
   (HL, day-care)
b. I met her at a dance in East LA.
   (HL, day-care)
c. she was one of the best dancers,
   I met her in East LA.
   (HL, day-care)

EXAMPLE 4
a. I don't hardly see him anymore,
   that is a big part of my life that has to be tried
   out.
   (VH, day-care)
b. I'm not good at writing you know,
   correspondence.
   neither of us really worked at it hard enough,
   I don't see him any more and that is such a
   part of my life.
   (VH, day-care)

EXAMPLE 5
a. I was married to an Italian,
   he was a whisky fiend.
   (AM, day-care)
b. my husband used to drink heavily,
   he was a whisky fiend.
   (AM, day-care)

EXAMPLE 6
a. my father was in charge of the saw mills,
   that dealt with timber and lumber.
   (AM, day-care)
b. my father was in charge of the saw mills,
   he used to cut lumber.
   (AM, day-care)
c. he worked for the saw mills,
   cut lumber and timber, y'know.
   (AM, day-care)

FIG. 6.1. Repeated chunks of talk in AD discourse.

constitute this chunk. For the purposes of this study, cognitive links or connections between events in a bound unit will be established in terms of the following:

1. *Adjacency*: Idea Y and idea X occur in conjunction, with idea X sometimes preceding Y, or with Y sometimes preceding X.
2. *Repetition*: The X–Y unit is repeated at least twice in the talk.

I take segments of at least two topically related lines as the minimal unit of analysis. That is, these segments have to meet the preceding criteria to be considered bound. Segments in Fig. 6.1 illustrate this:[5]

---

[5]These segments are drawn from the entire data pool.

Specific bits of information, in these examples have been linked together. They get repeated over and over again at different points in their respective narratives with little or no variation. The repetition in the three instances in Example 1 show how Ellie has chunked together information about her father's remarriage and her stepmother's dislike of her. Likewise, we see that Tina associates her father's dying of tuberculosis with the "trenches in France." In Example 6, AM associates her husband to his drinking habits ("My husband was a heavy drinker/he was a whisky fiend"), whereas HM has unitized information about where he met his wife ("I met her in East LA/I met her at a dance"). Implicit in these unitized chunks of information are the connections the tellers have established between events and the sense they have made of these different event schemas.

SEQUENCES OF EVENTS BEING BOUND IN ELLIE'S TALK

Whereas the previous section calls attention to ways in which bits of information have gotten bound, this section calls attention to ways in which entire sequences of events (more than two) have been unitized. I illustrate this point with three segments that Ellie repeats at least twice in our interaction. In Fig. 6.2, Examples 7 and 8 are about how she came to California. Examples 9 and 10 in Fig. 6.3 are about her parents' divorce,

EXAMPLE 7
Oh my sister was in the movies for 21 years
and when *they called me up and said she was dying*,
and *I had to hurry up here*,
she died within two days after I got here.
so I thought there is no use going back,
because she had a lot of stuff,
when you are in the movies you have a lot of junk to get rid of.
so I stayed here and sold her things,
but she was the only relative I had left,
so I didn't like it too much.
because *she was in the movies*,
and *I worked in big hotels in Chicago*,
[..] so we didn't see each other too much.

EXAMPLE 8
Well, *my sister was in the movies here*,
and *when she was dying, they called to come right away*,
she only lived that day yet.
so *that's how come I came here*,
and dropped every thing I was doing,
I was working in big hotels.
and was the one that shows everbody the seats,
and what to do,
so I worked about ten years.

FIG. 6.2. How Ellie got to California.

EXAMPLE 9
*I was 3 years old, when they got
divorced,*
so *I went to an orphanage.*
stayed there for a while,
couple years.
[..] then *my father got remarried,
and my stepmother took one look at me
and she could kill me.*
first thing I talked to she hated me,
so I stayed out of her way.
I ran away when I was 13,
I went to stay with my girl friend's mother,
she took me in.
she said "I know how you feel/I was brought up the
same way as you."
my dad couldn't even look for me,
'cause he had his own business and couldn't leave.
and he was very upset,
when I ran off,
but I never told him.
'cause she used to beat me up,
[...] *stepmother* [...] *she was* [.] *like that,
like that* [gesturing],
so *I just ran away.*
stayed at my girl friend's house,
her mother was very nice.

EXAMPLE 10
Oh well my childhood,
*my folks got divorced
when I was 3 years old,*
and *I was brought up in an
orphanage.*
and then my father got remarried,
'cause they told him so long,
as he had a good business,
he was a master tailor,
he could take care of his daughter.
and her let her grow up,
[slight pause/laughs] in an
orphanage.
*so he got remarried,
and she took one look at me,
and hated the sight of,
me the wife.*
so I stayed home for 2 years,
and I ran away again [laughs],
she said "*I could stand any
girl but YOUR daughter,*
I kept hearing that.
I smile.
...
so one day I ran away,
and was working within an hour,
changed my last name,
so they're lookin' for me,
they couldn't find my me.

FIG. 6.3. Ellie's childhood.

whereas 11 and 12 in Fig. 6.4 are about advice she gives her daughter. I have highlighted those utterances (including variations) that get repeated.

Ellie's bound talk demonstrates links she has made between particular event schemata. Her move to California, for instance, is strongly associated with her sister's dying (Examples 7 and 8). Also bound into this unit are utterances about their jobs: her sister being in the movies while Ellie "worked in big hotels." Her repetition of this sequence of events highlights the order in which she has encoded these event schemata: In both instances, she talks first of her sister being in the movies, then of the latter's dying and her own "hurrying up here," followed by the autobiographical fact about "working in big hotels." Likewise, her segment about her parents' divorce demonstrates strong connections she makes with her stepmother and orphanage (Examples 9 and 10). This sequence of event schemata also follows a certain order: the fact that she was 3 years old when her "folks got divorced," followed by her going to an orphanage, followed by her father's remarriage and her stepmother "hating the sight" of her, followed by her running away. Her segments on her advice to her daughter (Examples 11 and 12) also demonstrate conjunction between certain utterances: In this case, they specifically associate her daughter's marriage with "having fun" while she can.

These frozen segments of talk, with their terminal, tightly drawn boundaries, would lead one to believe that they would not be easily integrated into an ongoing life story (Strauss's, 1992, study explores this). However, I believe that these bound segments, complete and closed as they may seem, can be integrated when understood in terms of the teller's overall interpretive schemas, as subdivisions of an overall framework.

EXPLANATORY STATEMENTS AND THE ORGANIZATION OF EVENT SCHEMA

Before establishing how the events in Ellie's life story get connected to her overall interpretive schema, I briefly discuss how the events themselves get connected to each other. Researchers such as D'Andrade (1992) and Wyer and Gordon (1984) proposed a hierarchical organization of schema, and they demonstrate this with an "eating at the restaurant" script. Figure 6.5 is a simplified version of Wyer and Gordon's model.

According to Wyer and Gordon, the most general schema about eating at a restaurant may be encoded in terms of different subschemas: entering the restaurant, eating, and leaving. Each of these subschemas (eating, for

EXAMPLE 11	EXAMPLE 12
She's in Texas now ...,	She didn't have to get married or anything like that,
she's about 18,	
engaged to be married.	I told her "make sure you marry the right one,'
I told her "don't rush it/ *have the fun before you,*	*'cause after a while you'll feel like you missed out on something so have the fun*
get married"	*before you get married,*
'cause after a while you feel you could have had more things to do.	unless you have to commit.
marriage takes a lot out of you.	"Ma, how can you say a thing like that?"
	I said "I'm just telling you ahead of time..*have fun while you can."*

FIG. 6.4. Ellie's advice to her daughter.

EATING AT A RESTAURANT

```
         Entering              Eating                Leaving
       ┌────┴────┐         ┌─────┴─────┐          ┌────┴────┐
   greet waiter  go to table  order meal  eat meal  pay check  leave tip
                          ┌──────┴──────┐
                   waiter brings menu  decide meal
```

FIG. 6.5. Schemas and subschemas in a hierarchical model.

instance) consists of several specific acts (asking for the menu, reading it, deciding what to eat, telling the waiter, etc.) These specific acts, in turn, can be further subdivided. They propose that events and subevents, demonstrated in Fig. 6.1, are "tagged" to denote their temporal location at each level of the hierarchy.[6] Such a hierarchical model can, I believe, be applied to the encoding of autobiographical information as well. In terms of life stories, different life events and subevents get connected to each other and to the teller's overall schema. Some of these connections are evident through certain explanatory statements that a teller makes. At a general level, explanatory statements are the narrative equivalent of what Tracy (1983) referred to as "issue" in her *issue–event* concept in interactions, a term that she defines as a "general statement of principle, feeling, or belief" (p. 321). Like issues, explanatory statements are also statements that indicate principle, feeling, or belief. However, specific criteria are needed by which to identify such statements in discourse. In the present study such statements are evident in one or more of the following ways:

1. When the teller steps out of the narrative world and directly addresses the listener/audience
2. When the teller makes a statement—often toward the end of the narrative—that sums up her view about the event
3. When the teller makes a statement that indicates how the recounted narrative supports her view about herself.

---

[6]Wyer and Srull (1994) maintained that representations of events at the most general level (i.e., entering the restaurant, eating and leaving) "may carry tags that denote the general point in the sequence at which they occur (e.g., 'early,' 'middle,' 'late,' p. 107)." Representations at more specific levels may carry not only these tags, but also a tag that denotes their temporal position among those within the more general event.

Statements such as these render narrative discourse meaning-based in that they require the teller to "attend to deeper, more elaborate meanings" (Ellis et al., 1994) in the evolving life story. That is, the speaker has to be cognitively involved in and aware of several factors simultaneously (the audience's needs, contextualizing information, connecting life events) in such a way as to establish a point about herself (Linde, 1993; Ramanathan-Abbott 1993, 1994, 1995a). As we see later, explanatory statements in Ellie's lifestory reflect her relative control over these factors: They explain the links she has established between different life events and the overall meaning she has made of them.

A SCHEMATIC ANALYSIS OF ELLIE'S LIFE STORY

I begin with the following opening segment of Ellie's life story, variations of which are repeated 3 times during our interaction.

>EXAMPLE 13
>>*My sister was in the movies* for 21 years,
>>and when they called me up and said she was dying,
>>and I had to hurry up *here*.
>>she died within two days after I got here,
>>but she was the only relative I had left,
>>*so I didn't like it too much.*
>>because she was in the movies,
>>and I worked in big hotels in *Chicago*,
>>[..] *so we didn't see each other too much.*

The italicized utterances in this bound segment demonstrate Ellie's feeling *physically* distanced from her sister: Ellie's sister was in the movies in California while Ellie "worked in big hotels in Chicago." Her utterances "I didn't like it too much" and "We didn't see each other too much" emphasize the spatial separation. Her other bound narrative (repeated twice in our interactions) about her parents' divorce also captures this theme of distance; however, unlike this segment, the following segment calls attention to *emotional* distance.

>EXAMPLE 14
>>I was 3 years old, when they got divorced,
>>*so I went to an orphanage.*
>>stayed there for a while,
>>couple years.
>>[..] then *my father got remarried,*

> *and my stepmother took one look at me and she could kill me,*
> first thing I talked to she hated me.
> *so I stayed out of her way,*
> *I ran away* when I was thirteen,
> *I went to stay with my girl friend's mother,*
> she took me in.
> she said "I know how you feel/I was brought me up
> same way as you",
> *my dad couldn't even look for me,*
> 'cause he had his own business and couldn't leave,
> he was very upset when I ran off.
> but I never told him 'cause,
> she used to beat me up,
> [...] stepmother [...] she was [.] like that like that (gesturing),
> *so I just ran away.*
> stayed at my girl friend's house,
> her mother was very nice,
> *I went to live with a relative I didn't even know I had.*

The italicized utterances here stress Ellie's sense of feeling rejected ("I went to an orphanage," " my father remarried," "my stepmother used to beat me," "I stayed out of her way," "I ran away," "my dad couldn't even look for me,") and displaced ("I went to live with a relative"). Toward the end of this segment, however, her explanatory statements convey the meaning she has made of these events.

> EXAMPLE 15
> I ... got married early,
> just to get away from bothering somebody.
> *I didn't like that part,*
> they're were very nice to me.
> but *I'm better on my own,*
> *so I am still wandering around,*
> *sometimes I'm here and then I'm there.*

Ellie's utterances, "I ... got married early/ ... to get away from bothering somebody," reinforce her rootlessness articulated earlier. These also feed directly into her explanatory statements (the italicized utterances). Her statements "I'm better on my own," and "I'm still wandering around" contribute to her view of herself as one who is physically and emotionally displaced and distanced.

We get a sense of both physical and emotional distance when Ellie talks about her daughter in the following bound segment.

> EXAMPLE 16
> V: what about your daughter? what was bringing her
>   up like?

E: Oh *she's in Texas now,*
and I guess she married this man,
since she got married *she doesn't answer my letter,*
or anything,
and I'm kinda worried.

A little later Ellie repeats this again.

EXAMPLE 17
She lives in Texas now,
I don't hear from her,
she doesn't answer my letters....

The "now" in "she's in Texas now" highlights physical distance inasmuch as it implies that although her daughter is presently in Texas, she was once with Ellie. The sense of emotional distance, though, comes through in the other italicized utterances: "I'm kinda worried," "she doesn't answer.... "

All of these bound events highlight Ellie feeling distanced. In the following section I call attention to unbound events that point to her maintaining distance, a theme particularly evident in her talk about men. In the following segment she talks about her husband's infidelity. Once again, the italicized utterances are the explanatory statements.

EXAMPLE 18
Tall and slim,
always in uniform,
ladies went wild over him.
I was married twice,
my first husband died,
he was always drunk.
tall and slim,
he had 3–4 wives,
all at the same time as me.
they weren't sure how many he had,
he married them all,
he had a lot of fun doing that you know [..].
so anybody asks me to get married,
"Oh go ask somebody else/don't ask me
I've already had it."
If I don't wanta go to bed or go out I'll stay
home, you know,
If I wanna go I'll go if I feel like it.
Don't have to answer to anyone,
But if you meet the right guy, it's supposed to work out fine.

After talking about how her husband's good looks attracted women ("tall and slim/always in uniform"), Ellie sketches out aspects of her marriage: her husband's drunkenness and his simultaneous marriage to several women.

These utterances lead to the high point of her narrative: "So anybody asks me to get married/ ... go ask somebody else ... I've already had it...." This high point meets the previously established criteria for explanatory statements and meaning-based narratives in two ways. First, it evidences her stepping out of her story world to justify her feelings to her listener ("If I don't wanta go to bed or go out, I'll stay at home, you know"). Second, it implicitly communicates her view about the event: She will do as she pleases so that she doesn't "have to answer to anyone."

Not only do these statements display her maintaining distance in that they point to her resistance to a committed relationship. They also inform her views about her second marriage as well.

EXAMPLE 19
V: what about your second marriage?
E: Well he was in outside Europe some place in the
found some other female,
and had a baby with her,
so I says "you better make a good father/get a
divorce and take care of the baby."

he said "let's forget about it and I'll
come move back in with you,"
I says "just take care of the baby you just had that's what you are
supposed to do,
I can find somebody else."
I'm not interested in getting married again,
just forget worrin about it,
just go out and have fun.

I didn't wanna be domesticated again.

Her second husband also "chased after other women." In this case her relationship did not work out because her husband had fathered a baby with another woman. After recounting how her husband wanted to move back in with her and her rejection of his proposition, she explains to her audience how the narrative informs her views about marriage ("I'm not interested in getting married"). She wishes to maintain her distance from men.

Ellie's resistance to committing to a long-term relationship is evident in her views about her boyfriends as well.

EXAMPLE 20
V: what's your boyfriend like?
E: Which one?
V: oh, how many do you have?
E: [laughs}
V: maybe that's the question I need to ask,

E: well it depends on what day,
one of them has Saturday off,
and the other has Wednesday off,
I told them I'd go with both,
he says "both of us?"
I say "yes, *I'm not interested in one*" [laughs].

Ah, one called me a bigamist,
and the other said I was man crazy,
I say "I don't think so/other wise I would be married otherwise."

I said "you could ask me to go to bed with you,
but ask somebody else,
I'm not the type."

and if they were vulgar,
"go away ask somebody else/I don't go for
that stuff,"
and they say "what do you think, you are better than the rest?"
I says "I don't/I'm just worried about me/*I don't*
wanna end up like that,"
They thought I was kinda snooty,
I says "not really."

Once again we see Ellie voice her reluctance to get tied down to one particular relationship. She makes it clear that she has more than one boyfriend (to my question "What is your boyfriend like? Ellie's responded "Which one?"), and a little later explains this with "I'm not interested in just one." Her utterances "You could ask me to go to bed with you but ask somebody else ... I don't go for that stuff" imply that she sees sexual involvement as a kind of commitment. Her explanatory utterance, "I don't want to end up like that," underscores her reluctance to commit and renders her talk meaning-based.

Her advice to her daughter also displays this reluctance.

EXAMPLE 21
She didn't have to get married or anything like this,
I told her "make sure you marry the right one,"
'cause after a while you'll feel like to missed out on something.
so you should have the fun first,
before you get married.
unless you have to commit.
"Ma, how can you say a thing like that?"
I said "I'm just telling you ahead of time,
... *have fun while you can*."

Ellie's utterance "have fun while you can" is explanatory in that it voices her view about commitment and marriage. She offers me the same advice.

EXAMPLE 22
E: you single too?
V: ya
E: *have fun while you can.*

Marriage for Ellie is not fun because it could lead to feeling you "missed out on something;" it is better to maintain one's distance. In the following she talks about how she maintains her distance by sometimes pretending she is not Ellie.

EXAMPLE 23
I said "you could ask me to go to bed with you/but ask somebody, else/I'm not the type."

"well you look the type,"
I say "well that's nice"
I bought a wig,
and the next day I had a wig on.
and they say "aren't you Ellie?"
I says "no not today" [laughs].

She wears a wig and pretends she is not the type that men think she is. When I ask her what looking the "type" means, she explains,

they like somebody that's willing,

and Ellie, as we have seen, is not willing.

All of the preceding unbound segments (Examples 18, 19, 20, 21, 22, and 23) articulate, in part, the sense and meaning that Ellie has made about relationships: about not wanting to be domesticated again, about having several boyfriends at the same time, about not wanting to be committed to one, about dodging sexual propositions should they lead to commitment. In all, she voices her need to maintain distance. Her bound segments, though, (Examples 13, 14, 15, 16, and 17) evidence her feeling distanced. I would like to propose that these views—maintaining distance and feeling distanced—are subschemas that get subsumed under her larger interpretive schema of distance. The map in Fig. 6.6 illustrates this. The boxed segments in the map indicate bound events; the unboxed events represent unbound events.

The figure visually represents connections between Ellie's bound and unbound events and between events and her overall schema of distance. A sense-making device by which she understands and connects events of her past, this overall schema (realized in part through her explanatory state-

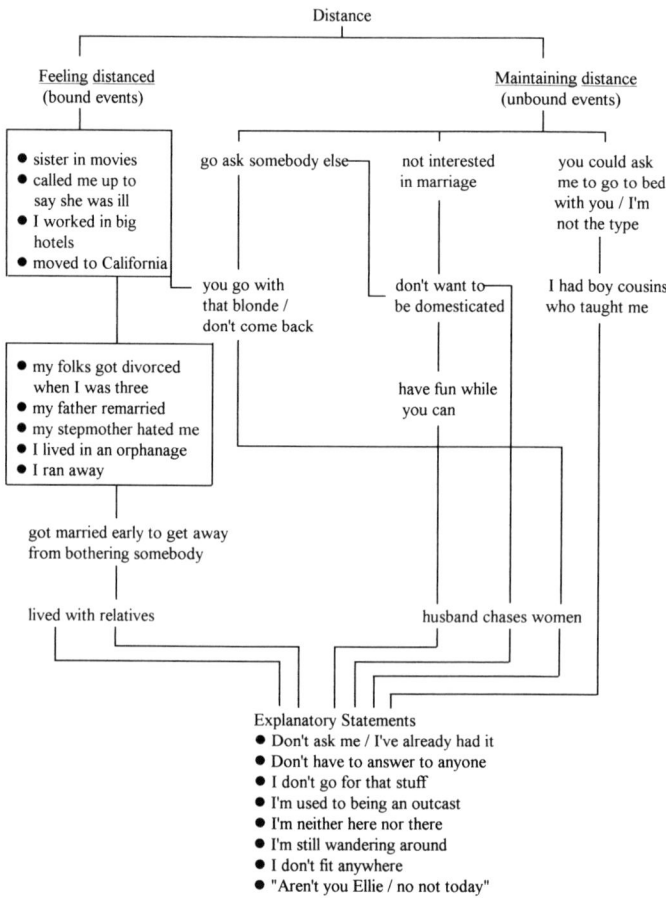

FIG. 6.6. A partial schematic map of Ellie's life story.

ments) is integral, not only to the way in which she sees her past and herself, but to rendering her discourse meaning-based. We are able to see remnants of this schema despite the ravages of the disease in her talk recorded a year and a half later. Before that, however, I present some background information on what transpired between the first recording and the second.

SOME NOTES ON ELLIE IN THE LATTER STAGES OF THE DISEASE

Shortly after her breakup with Tom, Ellie's deteriorating condition started to become more apparent. Now instead of hanging in bars, Ellie took to picking up men from the streets. Although her friends tried to keep her indoors, it was not always easy. One night she was accosted by the police for alleged prostitution and was locked up in jail. By the time authorities determined which day-care center Ellie attended, she already had been incarcerated about a week. When a caretaker from the day-care center went to pick her up, Ellie was found to have bruises around her eyes and legs. Exactly how she got them is not known.

Ellie was given a medical examination the day she was released from jail, after which she was diagnosed as having pneumonia. After being released from the hospital she was admitted to a convalescent home, which, according to one day-care caretaker, is a place "you are sent when you are sent to die." Her caretaker at that point had been in the process of finding other boarding arrangements for her. Members of the apartment complex in which she used to live did not want her back because "she was too much of a mess": She had lost control over her stool and bladder movements and, according to them, become an embarrassment.

She does not have much of a life in the convalescent home. She has much less interaction there (in fact almost none at all) than she did at the day-care center. She is strapped to a wheel chair because she is "too much of a liability." Because she was not allowed to walk after her surgery and because nobody encouraged her to, Ellie believes she cannot walk. She is afraid to try and needs a lot of cajoling to take a few steps. She still comes to the day-care center, transported by one of the vans, where she is made, for a few minutes each day, to exercise her legs.

These events have undoubtedly exacerbated Ellie's condition, and her rating by the aides at the day-care center dropped from "good" to "chair." It was around this time that I recorded her for the second time, and as we shall see, she is no longer able to narrate. The segments I use in the following section are drawn from this conversation.

EVIDENCE OF ELLIE'S INTERPRETIVE SCHEMA IN THE LATER STAGES OF ALZHEIMER'S DISEASE

Compared to her talk in our first interaction, Ellie's talk in the second recording seems more text-based. Villaume et al. (1989) defined text-based discourse as that which is "marked by simpler and more frequent speaking turns" that develop topics to a lesser extent because of "heavy reliance on passing moves, minimal replies and cohesive devices tying to the surface text of the interlocuter's most recent utterances" (p. 410). Ellie's talk at this time evidences some of these features. It also evidences discourse features associated with AD patients in the severe stages of the disease: incoherence, repetition, and semantic emptiness. Despite this, however, occasional utterances indicate that she has retained some of her schema of distance. In the following segment, I ask her about herself.

EXAMPLE 24
V: tell me about yourself Ellie
how did you come to California?
E: sometimes,
V: how did you come? have you always
been here?
E: well, *my mother and father don't live together anymore,*
so I just take it as it comes along.
V: ya
E: *I carry on by myself.*

Ellie's utterance, "My mother and father don't live together anymore," harks back to "My folks got divorced when I was three years old," and feelings of rejection and rootlessness that she articulated in her life story. In fact, soon after this, she explains: "I carry on by myself." This explanatory statement is similar to some of her previous explanatory utterances ("I'm on my own," "I'm used to being an outcast," "I'm still wandering around"). Like her earlier utterances, this one also voices her view about where she stands in relation to her past and herself.

We see her voicing a related sentiment of loneliness/rejection in the following instance. Several friends of Ellie's—other elderly folk—stop by and talk to Ellie when they see us in the courtyard, and it is after the last one has gone that the following exchange takes place.

EXAMPLE 25
V: you have a lot of friends here Ellie.
E: ya not too much,
V: quite a few people coming up to see how you are doing and how you
are feeling,
E: oh *I think they come to ask me about*
my husband,
they don't care about me.

Ellie had, in her earlier version of her life story, made mention at least twice of her handsome, wayward husband and the way he attracted women ("tall and slim/ ... ladies spoiled him"). Her utterance here, "I think they come to ask about my husband," recalls these previous utterances. Earlier we saw how her husband's infidelity got tied up with her maintaining her distance from men and not wanting to get committed again ("I'm not interested in getting married" ... /don't wanta be domesticated again"). This utterance ("They come to ask about my husband") echoes these connections. Although Ellie may no longer be able to remember the different details and events on which she bases this utterance, the fact that she still remembers women being drawn to her husband points to her retention of some of her schema. Likewise, her utterance, "they don't care about me," echoes her previously articulated sense of rejection and distance.

It is also evident that Ellie still maintains her distance by occasionally pretending she is not Ellie. An utterance in the following segment highlights this.

EXAMPLE 26
ME: are you really Ellie Jill?
E: *not really all depends on what I feel like,*
V: change your name whenever you want to, huh?
E: *ya right.*

When ME (male elderly) asks Ellie "Are you Ellie Jill?" Ellie's response is "Not really, all depends on what I feel like." Although none of the previous connotations (of not looking the "type") are evident in this statement, the fact that she still pretends she is not Ellie implies that she has retained some of her overall schema of distance.

We also see that her views about marriage have not changed. The following segment illustrates this

EXAMPLE 27
ME: you're a nice lookin chick, huh
E: I wasn't even aware of it.
ME: did you get married in between since I saw you?
E: oh no no no,
I'm not looking for trouble.

Ellie still associates marriage with "trouble." Her emphatic "no" (evident in the several times she says no: "Oh no no no") to ME's question and her utterance, "I'm not looking for trouble," lets us see that Ellie still views the idea of marriage distastefully.

DISCUSSION AND CONCLUSION

This chapter attempted to provide a relatively holistic picture of an AD patient's condition by juxtaposing a close analysis of her deteriorating discourse skills against her nonfacilitative social world. A point that resonates strongly from my field notes is that the social context happens to Ellie; she does little to shape it in turn. By the time of her second recording, she was not permitted to bathe, eat, or amuse herself.

Despite her progressively debilitating condition, exacerbated by her relatively unstable social environment, her discourse in our second recording evidences remnants of her overall interpretive schema that was discernable from the analysis of our first recording. As Cermak (1984) suggests, it is possible that with time and continued rehearsal, certain memories lose their *episodic* nature and become *semantic memories*, independent of temporal and spatial contexts. Whereas at one level Ellie's bound segments seem to have become decontextualized units, at another they are contextualized when understood in terms of her larger interpretive framework. Whereas previous research has called attention to ways in which repetition (in AD discourse) contributes to rendering patients' talk incoherent, this chapter attempted to display how repeated segments can reflect remnant linguistic skills that AD patients have retained. When understood in terms of an overall schema, these segments reflect "senseful," meaning-based connections that tellers make between certain events. The overall schema, then, becomes an overarching interpretive umbrella beneath which both bound and unbound events are subsumed and connected.

Bound talk in the data was identified in terms of two criteria: adjacency, (in which idea X and idea Y occurred in conjunction, regardless of order) and repetition (in which ideas were repeated at least twice in the talk). Taking the two-line segment as the minimal unit of analysis—in which a segment must have at least two related ideas—we saw evidence of bound talk in smaller segments (in which two ideas were adjacent and repeated) and in slightly larger segments (with several ideas comprising event sequences). Larger segments of bound talk pointed out in Ellie's discourse indicate that the teller had unitized chunks of events: Ellie clusters her ideas about her working in big hotels with her sister being in the movies and dying. Likewise, she connects her parents' divorce with her stepmother disliking her and her running away.

Ellie has established connections between these pieces of information in ways that are congruent with her overall view of herself. The analysis of Ellie's story reveals that, on the basis of her experiences, she has surmised certain things (both about the experiences themselves and about herself), that are partially realized in her explanatory statements, discourse features that render her life story meaning-based. Her views—about being an outcast, about "wandering around here and there," about being on her own—are all based on her life experiences: her running away when her father remarried, her stepmother disliking her, her wayward husbands, or men propositioning her. These events support the teller's explanatory statements, which, in turn, become ways by which the teller interprets these events. An ongoing cycle of events and views coloring each other, both together reinforce the teller's overall interpretive schema—of distance.

As these explanatory statements are based on a lifetime of events, many of which have probably been made sense of several times before, the overall interpretation of these events is not likely to change easily. We saw in Ellie's case that she retains some of her views despite the worsening of her disease, the increasing instability of her social world, and her deteriorating linguistic abilities. Although she no longer is able to remember the details of events or even the events themselves—evident in the relatively text-based nature of her discourse (minimal turns, unelaborated utterances and undeveloped topics)—she is able to recall certain utterances that can be recognized as throwbacks to an earlier schema.

Macro- and microanalyses such as the preceding enable us to see the parallel, yet invisibly intersecting tracks of a patient's language (in)abilities and (non)facilitative environments. The ethnographic details are meant to provide the backdrop against which the significance of the microanalysis is to be understood. The microanalysis permits us to view AD repetition, not as segments that contribute to meaninglessness in the patients' discourse, but as segments that capture, albeit in frozen ways, the teller's attempt at making sense of his or her life. Such an analysis shifts attention away from language breakdown, a notion commonly associated with Alzheimer discourse, to remnant language "wellness."

7

Some Implications and Conclusions

> Theorizing about the structure, forms, and rules of social action requires ... [a] type of narrative analysis that preserves the complex ordering of actions and reactions that constitute social reality ... [T]he story contains a sequence of socially meaningful acts without which it would not be a story; its analysis therefore provides the basis for a direct interpretation of a complex unit of social interaction, in comparison to the standard approach where such inferences are based on decontextualized bits and pieces.
>
> —*Elliot Mishler* (1986b)

A primary aim of the present volume has been to provide a complementary view toward understanding the deteriorating linguistic abilities of Alzheimer's disease (AD) patients. Instead of viewing "incoherence" in AD speech strictly in cognitive terms, (i.e., due to some malfunction in the brain) this study has attempted to show that the patient's inability to talk extensively and meaningfully is partially tied to audience turns and to the patient's social world. Lubinski (1991) mentions some ways in which the "perception of incompetence associated with dementia determines the social and communicative opportunities the individual will have and eventually the care that the individual will receive" (p. 142). Certainly, Ellie seemed to follow this route: When her rating fell from the "good" to the "chair" type, communicative opportunities were almost nonexistent. Although it is not this kind of classification that Lubinski is talking about, it is certainly applicable. Caregivers, as she points out, often segregate individuals in their "best interest," locking doors, isolating them from the world of activity, and restraining them to particular areas. As the ethnographic details in chapter 6 underscore, all of these are features remniscent of the operations at the day-care center that Ellie attended, where AD patients are housed in an enclosed area with their movements very closely monitored.

The care that Tina received contrasts sharply with Ellie's. Tina was cared for at home by her husband, had family that visited her every few months, went to a day-care center that encouraged language use, and generally operated, until quite recently (2 months ago), in a social environment that afforded her meaningful contexts within which to interact. She retained her mild to moderate condition for about 5 years. Although I am unable to provide direct evidence linking her relatively more stable condition to her relatively stable environment (or for linking Ellie's rapidly deteriorating state to her generally unstable social world for that matter), one cannot help speculating that her facilitative world contributed, to some extent, to stabilizing her condition.

Ellie's relatively accelerated deterioration may be partially because of her learning her helplessness. (Lubinski, 1991; Peterson, Maier, & Seligman, 1993). Research on the "learned helplessness" syndrome suggests not only that dementia is a "real change in cognitive, emotional and communicative behavior, but [that it] is also a learned behavior emanating from the perceptions of those in the environment" (Lubinski, 1991, p. 142). Among other features, it is marked by an *inappropriate passivity* (Peterson et al., 1993) that patients seem to acquire when they internalize their sense of incompetence from messages they get from their social world." When demented persons perceive that their responses are futile, they stop responding" (p. 142). The patient is diagnosed as having dementia, which in turn determines the kind of care and communication he or she receives. This care and communication carries with it "metamessages" (Tannen, 1987) of incompetence that the patient then internalizes. Figure 7.1 is a visual representation of this vicious cycle.

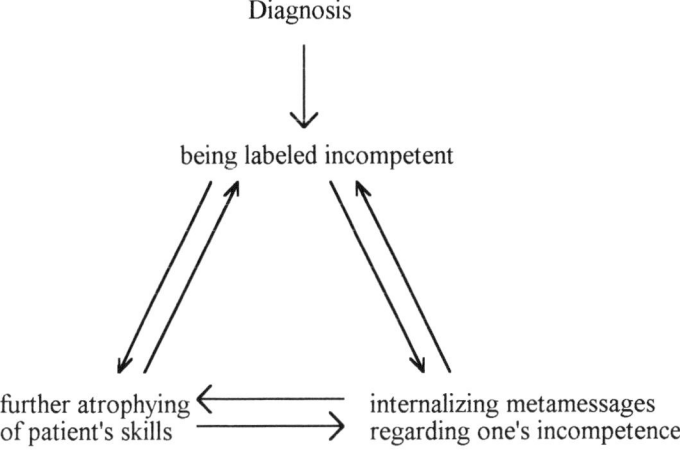

FIG. 7.1. Cycle of learned helplessness. Adapted from data from Lubinski (1991).

In the "best interest" of the patient, the caregiver begins to assume responsibility for the patient's moves. According to Lubinski (1991), the demented individual receives *outcome cues* that include responses from others in the environment concerning the inadequacy of patient's performance.

> Significant others in the environment do not expect the individual to perform capably and provide direct feedback concerning both actual and potential failure. For example, caregivers may verbally or nonverbally tell a person that they cannot perform a task, may repeatedly correct communication that is in error, or limit communication opportunities. (p. 144)

This "taking over" for the patient is partially illustrated in N's interaction with Tina—evident in his repair utterances, his inability to hear her narrative cues, his interpretation of shared events being the "correct" ones—in which he unconsciously assumes that she needs help retrieving and selecting events from her past. As we noted, this explains why is he able only to engage her in recognition instead of recall.

We can see evidence this in the second interaction between Ellie and myself as well. The following are some segments in which I seem to be engaging her only in recognition.

EXAMPLE 1
I:	I remember the last time I talked to you,	35
	it was almost a year ago, right?	36
	you ahm you used to talk to me a lot about your sister,	37
	you used to tell me that you lived in Chicago once,	
	is that right?	38
E:	ya quick fast thing going here going there more or less.	39

EXAMPLE 2
V:	*I remember you used to talk to me about your marriage Ellie,*	51
	you said you were married to an air force sergeant once,	52
E:	ya that's right my you got a good memory,	53
	it's more than I have.	54
V:	so tell me about that Ellie	55
E:	I'm too busy.	56
V:	that's what you said	57
E:	so I like to keep busy so I don't,	58
V:	what do you do to occupy your time?	59
E:	I'm too busy to even be bothered.	60

EXAMPLE 3
V:	*you told me your sister was in the movies,*	40
E:	that's right, hey you've got a good memory.	41
V:	you told me all this Ellie, *you used to be real fond of your sister right?*	42

E:	still am,	43
V:	where's she now?	44
E:	Chicago.	45
V:	*ya? I thought you were the one in Chicago and she was the one here*	46
E:	ya we changed.	47

In each of the above segments, I, like N, am holding up the events of Ellie's past for her to recognize. All of the italicized utterances are event-specific, the way Nick's were—"You told me you lived in Chicago," "You were married to an air force sergeant," "Your sister was in the movies"—with none of them eliciting extended talk from Ellie. A numerical count reveals that 10.4% of my turns (56 turns in all) in our second interaction were recognition-engaging turns. It is possible that, like N, my event-specific questions in segments such as the preceding can be seen to be motivated by my unconscious assumption that Ellie perhaps cannot recall and so needs help in reconstructing her past. Because I am aware of some of Ellie's past events, I too seem to be engaged in retrieving and selecting events for her to recognize.

Intertwined with outcome cues are what Lubinski (1991) called *situational cues* that contribute to the learned helplessness syndrome. These are cues sent out to the patient by the environment that he or she is no longer expected to act responsibly or competently. Even the fact that demented individuals are closely watched to prevent potential harm, embarrassment, or difficult situations is an indication that they are not expected to act responsibly (Miller & Norman, 1979). We saw evidence of such cues in Ellie's case, starting with reduced opportunities at the day-care center, building up to her apartment members evicting Tom from her apartment, and then her finally being sent to a convalescent home.

The different continuity and discontinuity elements studied in the preceding chapters provide a sense of how particular types as well as particular positioning of audience-turns contribute to perpetuating the learned helplessness cycle or breaking it. We saw that turns such as affirmations, formulations, sustainers, and newsmarks help patients recall and keep interaction on track. We also saw that my turns facilitated extensive talk from the patients when it occurred toward the beginning of narrative segments, that they served as queries that "warmed them up" to the activity in which I was attempting to engage them. In contrast, interactions got derailed when my turns occurred toward the end of narrative segments. It is possible that my turns were interpreted as drastic topic changes to which patients were not able to adjust because they had just finished talking extensively about something else. Extended pauses likewise threatened our interactions. As we saw, these extended pauses seemed mainly to occur at TRP's when I did not take my turn in the interaction. Although this was deliberate on my part because I wanted the patients to keep talking, it was, in effect, derailing our interactions.

SOME METHODOLOGICAL IMPLICATIONS

Hamiliton (1994) calls attention to how previous psycholinguistic research has based assessments about the communicative abilities of these patients on speech elicited in a rigid interview setting. She cites Bayles (1979) in which a patient is asked to talk about a common subject such as a button and then repeat what the researcher says. She illustrates her points with the following segment.

EXAMPLE 4
E: Is it very big?
P: No, it's not very big. No it's not very big
E: What color is it?
P: Well, it's not black, and it's not exactly brown, I don't know what it is
E: Say, "A little girl found a penny"
P: A little girl tore her heart
E: Say, "The president lives in the White house."
P: The horse lives bright horse drawers.
(cited in Hamilton, 1994, pp. 165–166)

Hamilton maintains that "the drill-like atmosphere" of this segment inhibits the patient from undertaking "any communicative initiative or attempt to attain any communicative goal" (p. 166). Patients have to feel the need to communicate or at least be encouraged to talk about things in which they are interested As the evidence in this study indicates, creating naturalistic settings that reduce test-related anxiety seem more likely to generate extensive and meaningful talk from patients. This was one reason why the present study focused on self-narratives. Although there is no direct evidence that patients are more likely to be communicative when asked about themselves rather than a button, the fact that most of the patients were able to engage in at least some recall suggests that they did not find talking about their pasts too problematic.

Another methodological implication has to do with subjecting the researcher's role to close analysis, what I referred to in chapter 1 as reflexive researching. As we saw, turning the critical lens on my contribution to patient talk revealed ways in which *I* was inhibiting patients from engaging in recall. This notion of reflexivity or "bending back on itself" has been addressed by Steir (1991), who maintains that reflexivity is a circular process that "unfolds as a spiraling" allowing multiple perspectives (p. 2). Such a view allows one not only to see all research as socially constructed but also to see, how the researchers motives and assumptions inform the interactions. Such a view has the potential of making us researchers uncomfortably aware that there may be in a sense no objective reality, that we bring our biases to the analyses of anything, and that any conclusion(s) we derive are always subjective (for a fuller discussion see Gergen & Gergen, 1991; Jorgenson, 1991). In this sense then, the interpretations offered in this study say as much about me as researcher as they do about the communicative (in)abilities of Alzheimer patients.

SOME INTERVENTIONIST STRATEGIES

Basing my discussion partially on the analyses of the previous chapters, I now turn to addressing some language-related interventionist strategies that can be used in the training of caregivers of AD patients. Because communicative dysfunction is a universal outcome of the disease, as much psycholinguistic research has found, mitigating the communicative conditions of these patients may, to some extent, contribute to stabilizing the patients' condition. The following are some ways by which we as audiences/caregivers can improve communication with patients who are in the mild to moderate stages of the disease and whose hold on language is still relatively strong.

Developing Audience/Caregiver Skills

Developing Listening Skills. Learning to listen to AD patients carefully to where we can "hear" their cues to talk or narrate is one way of encouraging them to talk extensively about what they care about. Bohling (1991) points out ways in which caregivers unable to hear patient signals cannot enter into patients' frames. Instead, they make the patient adjust to the frames they set, as illustrated by the following segment.

```
EXAMPLE 5
P:  This is known as polish, otherwise may be              1
    something                                              2
C:  tell me are you looking forward to our party?          3
P:  yes, what day is it?                                   4
C:  That is 1 week from today. Today's                     5
    Wednesday                                              6
P:  Really? That's when they ...                           7
C:  Do you know what day it is today?                      8
```

P:	Today. lets see. What was the question you said?	9 10
C:	Today is Wednesday. What would ...	11
P:	Wednesday? The best one is uh ...	12
C:	It will be one week ...	13
P:	One week after that? So that's all you have? You have that plus the one that you took.	14 15
C:	*And what's the date of the party? Wednesday. What date?*	16 17
P:	You know too much	18
C:	the 20th	19
P:	the 20th?	20
C:	*Do you want me to give you an invitation?*	21

(Bohling, 1991, p. 58, italics added)

This patient (P) sets the frame by talking about polish, but the caregiver does not enter her frame by furthering talk about it. Instead we see him or her set another frame with "Tell me are you looking forward to our party?" The patient then adjusts to this frame (Lines 4 and 6) when the caregiver changes it again in Line 8 ("Do you know what day it is today?"). Once again the patient adjusts to the new frame until the caregiver decides to change it yet again in Line 16, this time back to the earlier frame about the party. We see the caregiver change frames for the fourth time in Line 21 despite the patient's frustrated comment in Line 18 ("You know too much"). Bohling (1991) points out that "sensitive listening and partial entry into the patient's frame may be an effective listening response that will prevent [patient] anxiety from building to critical levels" (p. 262).

The caregiver's talk in the above segment is remniscent of N's talk with Tina in which he is unable to hear her narrative cues. The following segment is a reprint of a segment discussed in chapter 5.

EXAMPLE 6

N:	What's been happening at CAPS (the day-care center) lately?	1
T:	Oh not much, I uh we did we sort of did, [...]	2
N:	*what's happening with Francis? Is she still bothering you?*	3
T:	Ya she did, she took away my my ... she's horrible,	4
N:	*is she still taking away your stuff? She's always taking away your things, I wonder if she took away your coat, remember you'd lost your coat at the center?*	5 6 7
T:	ya and and ah she tore she tore my paper/ I ah I was,	8

N:	What paper? were y'all drawing?	9
T:	no no we we were using sticks [crayons?] and the paper ah was in,	10
N:	What's her problem? I spoke to C [the manager of CAPS] about her and ...	

N's role in the above segment is similar to C's role in Example 5 in that he too sets and controls the frames and makes the patient adjust to them. By constantly "taking charge," caregivers may be unconsciously diminishing the patient's dignity and independence (Bohling, 1991). One reason for their doing so may be because they may have unconsciously assumed the incompetence of the patients. Making caregivers sensitive to patient cues and encouraging them to focus on the patients' remnant linguistic skills instead of assuming language deficits is one way of addressing this problem.

Learning to Ask Open-Ended Questions. As some of the data in the previous chapters pointed out, asking relatively general questions about the patients' day, or past, or views is more likely to elicit extended talk from them since they (the patients) have to bear the onus of retrieving and selecting information. The more the shared knowledge between caregiver and patient, the more difficult this is likely to be because the caregiver would have to fight the temptation of providing all the information to the patient. We saw in N's interaction with Tina and my interaction with Ellie that we were holding up events of the patients' past for them to recognize, and our questions were inhibiting them from engaging recall. These findings underscore the need of sensitizing caregivers and other interactants to ways in which their questions determine the extent of talk their patients are able to produce.

Monitoring One's Use of Continuity and Discontinuity Elements. As the analyses in chapters 3, 4, and 5 point out, continuity elements such as affirmations, newsmarkers, continuers, and sustainers serve to keep patient talk on track, thus facilitating recall. Likewise, discontinuity elements such as extended pauses and repair inhibit patients from engaging in extended turns. We also saw how the particular positioning of audience turns influenced whether patients were able to recall. On an average, patients seemed to be able to engage successfully in recall when my turns appeared toward the beginning of narrative segments as opposed to when they occurred toward the end of the narratives. Training caregivers first to "hear" the beginnings and ends of narrative sequences and then to recognize continuity and discontinuity elements in *their own* discourse would allow them to see how their contributions engage patients in particular activities such as recall, reminding and recognition.

Encouraging Spaced-Retrieval Life Stories

Encouraging patients at repeated time intervals to recall parts of their pasts has been proven useful. Referred to as the spaced-retrieval method (Landauer & Bjork, 1978), it was developed initially for memory-impaired people and has been adapted for AD patients with some success. On the basis of her close study of two AD patients diagnosed with very mild AD, Riley (1990) surmised that the spaced-retrieval technique led to fairly rapid learning. A major goal of the study was to see if the spaced-retrieval technique would be useful to the patient and caregiver in the home environment once the training sessions were completed. Toward this end, Riley had four weekly one hour training sessions with the caregiver of the patient as an active participant of the intervention team. Aspects that Riley included in her study were individually designed training programs, making caregivers a part of the research team, assigning homework, and doing long-term follow up (Riley, 1992).

Because one's memories and past are crucial to one's sense of self and identity, having AD patients recall parts of their pasts at spaced retrievals would enable them to preserve a relatively active sense of their past. Furthermore, having them do so with their primary caregivers would reduce performance-related anxiety that patients are likely to feel when being tested. Indeed, several reminiscence experts (e.g., Merriam, 1989; Schafer, 1994) maintain that there are several benefits to reminiscing about one's past, including helping the teller to preserve personal identity and self-esteem. Revere and Tobin (1980, 1981) believe that the act of dramatizing or mythicizing past events can help tellers to see the uniqueness of their pasts. Others call attention to the social and contextual aspects of reminiscing (David, 1990; Tarman, 1988), showing how making status claims can elicit positive responses from others (Marshall, 1980), how joint reminiscing can be an entertaining social activity (McMohan & Rhudick, 1964), and ways in which it helps to bridge connections between generations (Pincus, 1970). An interactional look at life stories enables one to see the kinds of events/experiences that the teller chooses to select and highlight, depending on who he or she is talking to and the kind of self the teller is trying to present. Tarman (1988) highlighted the importance of "controlling one's biography" (Schafer, 1994) and emphasized the importance of the social situation for successful reminiscing.

At what general stage in the caregiver's "career" could some of these interventionist strategies make a significant difference? Aneshensel et al. (1995) maintain that a typical caregiver's career consists of three stages: (a) role acquisition, which entails recognizing the need for the role and assuming its obligations; (b) role enactment, which involves the actual performance of role-related tasks within the home and/or in a long-term care facility; and (c) role disengagement when the caregiver's role has ceased, typically after the patient has passed on. Training caregivers who care for patients both at home and in long-term care facilities in ("career") Stages 1 and 2, but primarily at Stage 2, might stem the learned helplessness syndrome from setting in too early.

IN RETROSPECT

It is in the nature of academic inquiry that new knowledge is consolidated with previous findings, and the work presented in this study realizes this at least to some degree. However, this study is not without its shortcomings, and I touch on these briefly because they can have implications for future research. One implication concerns the gathering of the data. It can be recalled that Tina was recorded across settings and audiences, but that the remaining 15 patients were not. Knowing if all 16 patients evidenced differences in their abilities to engage in extended and meaningful talk across audiences and settings would have been useful because it would make my point about interactional variation that much stronger. Although it can be speculated that the chances of such variation are high, gaining actual numbers would have been more persuasive. Furthermore, such an analysis may have revealed systematic interactional features across similar audiences.

Another way in which this study falls short and one that future research could pursue is in tracing ways in which AD patients might schematically organize their life stories differently with different audiences. Would Tina's schema, for instance, be different with her husband than with me? It is difficult to hypothesize about this one. An intuitive speculation would suggest that she would organize her life stories differently with both of us.[1] However, given that the memories of patients can get predominantly frozen and bound (evidenced partly in the repetition in Ellie's talk), it is likely that their overall schemas may become frozen and bound, and that these would remain unchanged regardless of audience. Much would depend on how "involved" the *audience* is in life story construction. If the audience is as involved as N is—doing the retrieving and selecting of life events for Ellie—then it is more likely that the audience is going to make sense of the patient's past as opposed to the patient doing so by him or herself.

---

[1]Seeing that N was doing most of the recalling for her, one could argue that Tina's overall schema was being set by N, at least in that particular interaction.

Finally, examining interactions with AD patients who are from other ethnic groups and other economic levels would be useful inasmuch as it would, among other things, shed light on whether social environments and available linguistic and communicative opportunities would be very different across ethnic and minority groups. It would also shed light on cultural factors that influence caregiving attitudes and behaviors in these social groups.

A CLOSING NOTE

As can be expected, many of my views about AD patients and their families changed as my study progressed. When I began my work as a volunteer in senior day-care centers, I felt an enormous gap between myself and the patients until I began to get to know them and some of their family members. I was, before long, able to see them as individuals: Blanca danced to imaginary music, Boris played an imaginary guitar, and Gloria always got all her food over herself. Operating in the day-care centers several hours a week for several years allowed me some insight into the subculture of some of these places: the extremely routinized nature of everday chores that rendered each day like every other; the food was so bland you could not recall it. Lunches and breakfasts were the only changes in routine. It brought home to me the extreme importance of providing rich, stimulating environments—social settings and interactions—that would allow patients to use language in meaningfully, communicative ways. My views regarding methodology changed enormously as well; turning the critical lens on myself helped me realize how fallible I was as researcher, that the very things I found wrong in caregiver behavior were things I was guilty of. All of this has, if anything, humbled me and it is in this spirit of humility that I share this work.

References

Abelson, R. (1968). Computers, polls and public opinions—some puzzles and paradoxes. *Trans-Action, 5*(9), 20–27.

Alzheimer, A. (1907). Ubereine ei genartig erkrankunger himvinde. *Allgemenic Zeitschrift für Psychiatric, 64,* 146–148.

Anderson, J. R., & Bower, G. H. (1972). Recognition and retrieval processes in free recall. *Psychological Review, 79*(3), 97–123.

Anderson, J. R., & Bower, G. H. (1974). A propositional theory of recognition memory. *Memory and Cognition, 2*(3), 406–412.

Aneshensel, C., Pearlin, L., Mullin, J., Zarit, S., & Whitlatch, C. (1995). *Profiles in caregiving: The unexpected career.* San Diego: Academic Press

Appell, J., Keretz, A., & Fisman, J. (1982). A study of language functioning in Alzheimer's patients. *Brain and Language, 17,* 73–91.

Bartlett, F. C. (1932). *Remembering: A study in experimental psychology.* Cambridge, England: Cambridge University Press.

Bauman, R. (1986). *Story, performance and event.* Cambridge, England: Cambridge University Press.

Bayles, K. A. (1979). *Communication profiles in a geriatric population.* Unpublished doctoral dissertation, University of Arizona, Tucson.

Bayles, K. A. (1982). Language function in senile dementia. *Brain and Language, 16,* 265–280.

Bayles, K. (1984). Language and dementia. In A. Holland (Ed.), *Language disorders in adults: Recent advances* (pp. 209–244). San Diego, CA: College Hill Press.

Bayles, K. A. & Tomoeda, C. K. (1983). Confrontation naming impairment in dementia. *Brain and Language, 19,* 98–114.

Bayles, K., Tomoeda, C., & Kasniak, A. (1985). Verbal perseveration of dementia patients. *Brain and Language, 2,* 102–116.

Bennet-Kastor, T. (1978). *Utterance repetition and social development: A case study of Genie and her caregiver.* Unpublished doctoral dissertation, University of Southern California.

Biglan, A., Glaser, S., & Dow, M. (1980). *Conversational training for social anxiety: An evaluation of its validity.* Unpublished manuscript, University of Oregon.

Bloom, L, Rocisano, L., & Hood, L. (1976). Adult–child discourse: Development interaction between information processing and linguistic knowledge. *Cognitive Psychology, 8,* 521–522.

Bohling, H. (1991). Communication with Alzheimer patients: An analysis of caregiver listening patterns. *International Journal of Aging and Human Development, 33*(4), 249–267.

Brown, J. (1976). An analysis of recognition and recall and of problems in their comparison. In J. Brown (Ed.), *Recall and recognition* (pp. 1–35). London: Wiley.

Bruner, J., & Weisser, S. (1991). The invention of self: Autobiography and its forms. In D. Olson & N. Torrance (Eds.), *Literacy and orality.* Cambridge, England: Cambridge University Press.

Buckingham, H., Whitaker, H., & Whitaker, H. (1976). On linguistic perserveration. In H. Whitaker & H. Whitaker (Eds.), *Studies in neurolinguistics* (Vol. 4, pp. 329–352). New York: Academic Press.

Camp. C. J. (1988). In pursuit of trivia: Remembering, forgetting, and aging. *Gerontology Review*, 1, 37–42.
Chafe, W. (1974). Language and consciousness. *Language*, 50, 111–133.
Chafe, W. (1982). Integration and involvement in speaking, writing and oral literature. In D. Tannen (Ed.), *Spoken and written language: Exploring orality and literacy* (pp. 35–53). Norwood, NJ: Ablex.
Coulthard, M. (1977). *An introduction to discourse analysis*. London: Longman.
Carr, D. (1985). Life and narrator's art. In H. J. Silverman & D. Idhe (Eds.), *Hermeneutics and deconstruction* (pp. 108–121). Albany: State University of New York Press.
Casey, E. (1989). *Remembering: A phenomenological study*. Bloomington: Indiana University Press.
Cegala, D. (1981). Interaction involvement: A cognitive dimension of communicative competence. *Communication Education*, 30, 109–121.
Cermak, L. (1984). The episodic/semantic distinction in amnesia. In N. Butters & L. Squire (Eds.), *The neuropsychology of memory* (pp. 55–62). New York: Guilford Press.
Coupland N, Coupland, J., & Giles, H. (1991). *Language, society and the elderly: Discourse, identity and aging*. Oxford: Blackwell.
D'Andrade, R. (1992). Schemas and motivation. In R. D'Andrade & C. Strauss (Eds.), *Human motives and cultural models* (pp. 23–44). Cambridge: Cambridge University Press.
David, D. (1990). Reminiscence, adaptation and social context. *International Journal of Aging and Human Development*, 30, 175–188.
Denzin, N. (1989). *Interpretive biography*. Newbury Park: Sage
Ellis, D. (1996). Coherence patterns in Alzheimer discourse. *Communication Research*, 23(4), 472–495.
Ellis, D., Duran, R., & Kelly, L. (1994). Discourse strategies of competent communicators: Selected cohesive and linguistic devices. *Research on Language and Social Interaction*, 27, 145–170.
Eisensen, J. (1971). Therapeutic problems and approaches with aphasic adults. In L. E. Travis (Ed.), *Handbook of speech pathology and audiology*. New York: Appleton Century-Crofts.
Eisensen, J. (1973). *Adult aphasia: Assessment and treatment*. New York: Appleton Century-Crofts.
Ferrara, K. 1994. *Therapeutic ways with words*. NY: Oxford University Press.
Freeman, M. (1984). History, narrative, life-span developmental knowledge. *Human Development*, 27, 1–19.
Freeman, T., & Gathercole, C. (1966). Perseveration—the clinical symptoms—in chronic schizophrenia and organic dementia. *British Journal of Psychiatry*, 112, 27–32.
Gee, J. P. (1990). *Social linguistics and literacies: Ideology in discourses*. New York: Falmer Press.
Gee, J. P. (1992). *The social mind*. New York: Bergin and Garvey.
Gergen, K., & Gergen, M. (1991). Toward reflexive methodologies. In F. Steir (Ed.), *Research and reflexivity* (pp. 76–95). London: Sage.
Goldstein, K. (1948). *Language and language disturbances*. New York: Grune & Stratton.
Grudin, R. (1982). *The time and art of living*. San Francisco: Harper & Row.
Hamilton, H. (1994). *Conversations with an Alzheimer patient*. Cambridge: Cambridge University Press.
Heir, D., Hagenlocker, K., & Shindler, A. (1985). Language disintegration in dementia: Effects of etiology and severity. *Brain and Language*, 25, 117–133.
Heritage, J. (1984). *Garfinkel and ethnomethodology*. Cambridge Polity Press.
Heritage, J. (1985). Analyzing news interviews: Aspects of the production of talk for an overhearing audience. In T. van Dijk (Ed.), *Handbook of discourse analysis: Vol. 3. Discourse and dialogue* (pp. 95–117). London: Academic Press.

Heritage, J. (1988). Explanations as accounts: A conversation analytic perspective. In C. Antaki (Ed.), *Analyzing everyday explanation* (pp. 127–144). London: Sage.

Heritage, J., & Atkinson, M. (1984). *The structures of social action.* Cambridge: Cambridge University Press.

Hollingworth, H. (1913). Characteristic differences between recall and recognition. *American Journal of Psychology, 24,* 532–544.

Hunt, M. (1990). *Narrative in mild and moderate dementia of the Alzheimer type.* Unpublished manuscript, University of Southern California.

Hutchinson, J., & Jensen, M. (1980). A pragmatic evaluation of discourse communication in the normal and senile elderly in a nursing home. In L. Obler & M. Albert (Eds.), *Language and communication in the elderly* (pp. 59–73). Boston: Lexington Books.

Irigaray, L. (1973). *Le Langue Des Dements.* The Hague: Mouton.

Jefferson, G. (1978). Sequential aspects of story telling in conversation. In J. Schenkein, (Ed.), *Studies in the organization of conversational interaction* (pp. 219–248). New York: Academic Press.

Johnstone, B. (Ed.). (1987). An introduction: Perspectives on repetition. *Text, 7,* 205–214.

Jorgenson, J. (1991). Co-constructing the interviewer/Co-constructing family. In F. Steir (Ed.), *Research and reflexivity* (pp. 210–225). London: Sage.

Katzman, R. (1986). Alzheimer's disease. *New England Journal of Medicine, 15,* 964–793.

Katzman, R. (1985). Current frontiers in research on Alzheimer's disease. In V. L. Melnick and N. N. Dubler (Eds.), *Alzheimer's dementia: Dilemmas in clinical research* (pp. 1–11). Clifton, NJ: Humana Press.

Keenan, E. (1977). Making it last. Repetition in children's discourse. In L. Ervin-Tripp, & C. Mitchell-Kernan (Eds.), *Child's discourse* (pp. 125–138). NY: Academic Press.

Kempler, D. (1991). Language changes in dementia of the Alzheimer's type. In R. Lubinski (Ed.), *Dementia and communication: Research and clinical implications* (pp. 95–114). Philadelphia: Decker Publishing.

Kintsch, W. (1970). Models for free recall and recognition. In D. A. Norman (Ed.), *Models of human memory* (pp. 247–308). New York: Academic Press.

Kirshner, H., Webb, W., Kelly, M., & Wells, C. (1984). Language disturbance: An initial symptom of cortical degeneration and dementia. *Archives of Neurology, 41,* 491–496.

Kraeplin, E. (1919). *Dementia praecox and paraphrenia.* Huntington, NY: Krieger.

Labov, W. & Waletzky, J. (1966). Narrative analysis: Oral versions of personal experience. In J. Helm (Ed.), *Essays on the verbal and visual arts* (pp. 12–45). Seattle, WA: University of Washington Press.

Labov, W. & Waletzky, J. (1968). Narrative analysis: Oral versions of personal experience. In J. Helm (Ed.), *Essays on the verbal and visual arts* (pp. 12–45). Seattle, WA: University of Washington Press.

Landauer, T. & Bjork, R. (1978). Optimal rehearsal patterns and name learning. In M. Gruneberg, P. Morris, & R. Skyes (Eds.), *Practical aspects of memory* (pp. 625–632). London: Academic Press.

Lerner, G. H. (1989). Notes on overlap management in conversation: The case of delayed completion. *Western Journal of Speech Communication, 53,* 167–177.

Light, E., & Lebowitz, B. D. (Eds.). (1990). *Alzheimer's disease treatment and family stress.* New York: Hemisphere Publishing.

Linde, C. (1987). Explanatory systems in oral life stories. In D. Holland & N. Quinn (Eds.), *Cultural models in language and thought* (pp. 343–366). Cambridge: Cambridge University Press.

Linde, C. (1993). *Lifestories.* Oxford: Oxford University Press.

Linton, M. (1982). Transformations of memory in everyday life. In U. Neisser (Ed.), *Memory observed* (pp. 77–91). San Francisco: Freeman.

Lubinski, R. (Ed.). (1991). *Dementia and communication: Research and clinical implications*. Philadelphia: Decker Publishing.

Mandelbaum, J. (1989). Interpersonal activities in conversational storytelling. *Western Journal of Speech Communication, 53*, 114–126.

Marshall, V. (1980). *Last chapters: A sociology of aging and dying*. Monterey, CA: Brooks/Cole.

Martin, A., & Fedio, P. (1983). Word production and comprehension in Alzheimer's disease: The breakdown of semantic knowledge. *Brain and Language, 19*, 124–141.

McLaughlin, M., & Cody, M. (1982). Awkward silences: Behavioural antecedents and consequences of the conversational lapse. *Human Communication Research, 8*(4); 229–316.

McMohan, A, & Rhudick, P. (1964). Reminiscing in the aged: An adaptational response. *Archives of General Psychiatry, 10*, 292–298.

Meacham, J. (1994). Reminiscing as a process of social construction. In B. Harght & J. Webster (Eds.), *The art and science of reminiscing*. Washington, DC: Taylor and Francis.

Meacham, J. (1995). Reminiscing as a process of social construction. In B. Haight & J. Webster (Eds.), *The art and science of reminiscing* (pp. 37–48). Washington, DC: Taylor and Francis.

Merriam, S. (1989). The structure of simple reminiscence. *The Gerontologist, 29*: 761–767.

Miller, I. & Norman, W. (1979). Learned helplessness in humans: A review and attribution theory model. *Psychological Bulletin, 86*, 93–118.

Mishler, E. (1984). *The discourse of medicine: The dialectics of medical interviews*. Norwood, NJ: Ablex.

Mishler, E. (1986a). *Research Interviewing: Context and narrative*. Cambridge: Harvard University Press.

Mishler, E. (1986b). The analysis of interview–narratives. In T. R. Sarbin (Ed.), *Narrative psychology: The storied nature of human conduct* (pp. 233–255). New York: Praeger.

Myers, F. (1988). Locating ethnographic practice: Romance, reality, and politics in the outback. *American Ethnologist, 15*, 609–624.

Neisser, U. (1982). *Memory observed*. San Francisco: W. H. Freeman and Company.

Nicholas, M., Obler, and Helm-Estabrooks (1985). Empty speech in Alzheimer's disease and fluent aphasia. *Journal of Speech and Hearing Research, 28*, 405–410.

Nofsinger, R. (1991). *Everyday conversation*. Newbury Park: Sage.

Norman, D. (1968). Toward a theory of memory and attention. *Psychological Review, 75*, 522–536.

Obler, L. (1981). Review of *Le langue des dements* by Luce Irigaray. *Brain and Language, 12*, 375–386.

Ochs, E. (1979). Planned and unplanned discourse. In T. Givon (Ed.), *Discourse and syntax* (pp. 51–80). New York: Academic Press.

Peterson, C., Maier, S., & Seligman, M. (1993). *Learned helplessness*. New York: Oxford University Press.

Pincus, A. (1970). Reminiscence in aging and its implication for social work practice. *Social Work, 15*, 47–53.

Polkinghorne, D. (1988). *Narrative knowing and the human sciences*. Albany: State University of New York Press.

Radley, A. (1990). Artifact, memory and a sense of the past. In D. Middleton & D. Edwards (Eds.), *Collective remembering* (pp. 46–58). London: Sage.

Ramanathan–Abbott, V. (1993). An examination of the relationship between social practices and the comprehension of narratives, *Text, 13*, 117–141.

Ramanathan, V. (1995a). Narrative wellformedness in Alzheimer discourse: An interactional examination across settings. *Journal of Pragmatics, 23*, 395–419.

Ramanathan, V. (1995b). Schematic understanding: evidence from Alzheimer discourse. *Communication Theory, 5*(3), 224–247.

Ramanathan-Abbott, V. (1994). Interactional differences in Alzheimer discourse: an examination of AD speech across two audiences. *Language in Society, 23* (1), 31–58.

Ramanathan, V. (1996). *Triggering recall: an examination of self and other-reminding prompts in Alzheimer interactions.* Unpublished manuscript.

Reisberg, B. (1981). *A guide to Alzheimer's disease.* New York: The Free Press.

Revere, V., & Tobin, S. (1980, 1981). Myth and reality: The older person's relationship to his past. *International Journal of Aging and Human Development, 12*, 15–26.

Riley, K. (1990). *The application of a memory maintenance program with demented elderly and their caregivers.* Paper presented at the Cognitive Aging Conference, Atlanta, GA.

Riley, K. (1992). Bridging the gap between researchers and clinicians: Methodological perspectives. In R. West & J. Sinnot (Eds.), *Everyday memory and aging*, (pp. 182–189). New York: Springer-Verlag.

Ripich, D. & Terrell, B. (1988). Patterns of discourse cohesion and coherence in Alzheimer's disease. *Journal of Speech and Hearing Disorders, 53*, 8–15.

Ross, M., & Buehler, R. (1994). On authenticating and using personal recollections. In N. Schwartz & S. Sudman (Eds.), *Autobiographical memory and the validity of retrospective accounts* (pp. 55–69). New York: Springer–Verlag.

Rumelhart, D. (1980). Schemata: The building blocks of cognition. In R. J. Spiro, B. C. Bruce, and W. F. Brewer (Eds.), *Theoretical issues in reading comprehension: Perspectives of cognitive psychology, linguistics, artificial intelligence and education* (pp. 33–58). Hillsdale: NJ: Lawrence Erlbaum Associates.

Rutter, M. (1966). Behavioural and cognitive characteristics of a series of psychotic children. In J. Wing (Ed.), *Early childhood autism: Clinical, educational and social aspects* (pp. 120–135). London: Pergamon Press.

Sabat, S. (1991). Turn-taking, turn-giving, and Alzheimer's disease: A case study in conversation. *Georgetown Journal of Languages and Linguistics, 2*, 161–175.

Sacks, H. (1974). An analysis of the course of a joke's telling in conversation. In R. Bauman & J. Scherzer (Eds.), *Explorations in the ethnography of speaking* (pp. 337–353). Cambridge: Cambridge University Press.

Sacks, H., Schegloff, E. A., & Jefferson, G. (1973). A simplest systematics for the organization of turn-taking in conversation. *Language, 50*, 696–735.

Schafer, D. (1994). *Reminiscence and nursing home life.* New York: Garland Publishing.

Schank, R. (1980). *Dynamic memory.* Cambridge: Cambridge University Press.

Schank, R. (1982). *Dynamic memory.* Cambridge: Cambridge University Press.

Schank, R., & Abelson, R. (1977). *Scripts, plans, goals and understanding.* Hillsdale, NJ: Lawrence Erlbaum Associates.

Schegloff, E. (1982). Discourse as an interactional achievement: Some uses of "uh-huh" and other things that come between sentences. In D. Tannen (Ed.), *Analyzing discourse: Text and talk* (pp. 71–93). Washington, DC: Georgetown University Press.

Schegloff, E., Jeffersen, G., & Sacks, H. (1977). The preference for self correction in the organization of repair in conversation. *Language, 53*, 361–382.

Schneck, M. K., Reisberg, B., & Ferris, S. H. (1982). An overview of current concepts of Alzheimer's disease. *American Journal of Psychiatry, 19*, 165–1287.

Schwartz, M. F. Martin, O., & Saffran, E. (1979). Dissociations of language function in dementia: A case study. *Brain and Language, 7*, 227–306.

Sherman, E. (1991). *Reminiscence and self in old age.* New York: Springer Publishing Company.

Steir, F. (1991). (Ed). *Research and reflexivity*. London: Sage.
Strauss, C. (1992). What makes Tony run? Schemas as motives reconsidered. In R. D'Andrade & C. Strauss (Eds.), *Human motives and cultural models* (pp. 197–224). Cambridge: Cambridge University Press.
Stubbs, M. (1983). *Discourse analysis*. Chicago: University of Chicago Press.
Swihart, A., & Prizzolo, F. (1988). The neuropsychology of aging and dementia: Clinical issues. In H. Whitaker (Ed.), *Neuropsychological studies of non-focal damage* (pp. 1–60). New York: Springer-Verlag.
Tannen, D. (1982). Oral and literate strategies in spoken and written narratives. *Language, 58, 1*, 1–21.
Tannen, D. (1987). Repetition in conversation as spontaneous formulaicity. *Text, 7*(3), 215–243.
Tannen, D. (1987). *That's not what I meant*. New York: Ballantine Books.
Tarman, V. (1988). Autobiography: The negotiation of a lifetime. *International Journal of Aging and Human Development, 27*, 171–191.
Tonkin. E. (1992). *Narrating our pasts*. Cambridge, England: Cambridge University Press.
Tracy, K. (1983). The issue–event distinction: A rule of conversation and its scope condition. *Human Communication Research, 9*, 320–334.
Tulving, E. (1976). Ecphoric process in recall and recognition. In J. Brown (Ed.), *Recall and recognition* (pp. 37–73). London: Wiley.
Ulatowska, H., Allard, L., Donnell, A., Bristow, J., Haynes, S., Flower, A., & North, A. (1988). Discourse performance in subjects with dementia of the Alzheimer's type. In H. Whitaker (Ed.), *Neuropsychological studies of non-focal brain damage* (pp. 108–131). New York: Springer-Verlag.
Villaume, W., Jackson, J., & Schouten, T. (1989). Issue–event extensions and interaction involvement: Text-based and meaning-based discourse strategies. *Human Communication Research, 3*, 195–213.
Watson, L., & Watson-Franke, M. B. (1985). *Interpreting life histories: An anthropological inquiry.*, NJ: Rutgers University Press.
Weimann, J. (1977). Explication and test of a model of communicative competence. *Human Communication Research, 3*, 195–213.
Wyer, R., & Gordon, S. (1984). The cognitive representation of social information. In R. Wyer & T. Srull (Eds.), *Handbook of social cognition* (pp. 73–150). Hillsdale, NJ: Lawrence Erlbaum Associates.
Wyer, R. S., & Srull, T. K. (1980). The processing of social stimulus information: a conceptual integration. In R. Hastie, T. Ostrom., E. Ebbesen, R. Wyer, D. Hamilton, & D. Carlston (Eds.), *Person Memory: Cognitive basis for social perception*. Hillsdale, NJ: Lawrence Erlbaum Associates.
Wyer, R. S., & Srull, T. K. (1984). *Handbook of Social Cognition*. Hillsdale, NJ: Lawrence Erlbaum Associates.

Author Index

A

Abbott, V., 2, 98, 104
Abelson, R., 90, 95, 96, 98
Ailes, H., 12, 84, 95, 96
Allard, L., 5, 90, 97
Alzheimer, A., 2, 3
Anderson, J. R., 18
Aneshensel, C., 124
Appell, J., 3, 5

B

Bartlett, F. C., 12
Bauman, R., 21
Bayles, K. A., 2, 3, 4, 17, 97, 120
Bennett-Kastor, T., 96
Biglan, A., 61
Bjork, R., 124
Bloom, L., 58
Bohling, H., 121, 122, 123
Bower, G. H., 18
Bristow, J., 5, 90, 97
Brown, J., 17
Bruner, J., 11, 13, 14, 70
Buckingham, H., 96
Buehler, R., 13

C

Carr, D., 30
Casey, E., 1
Cegala, D., 97
Cermak, L., 114
Chafe, W., 60, 98
Cody, M., 61, 62
Coulthard, M., 60
Coupland, J., 12, 84
Coupland, N., 12, 84

D

D'Andrade, R., 9, 90, 102

David, D., 124
Donnell, A., 5, 90, 97
Dow, M., 61
Duran, R., 89, 90, 97, 104

E

Eisensen, J., 96
Ellis, D., 3, 90, 91, 97, 104

F

Fedio, P., 4
Ferrara, K., 26
Ferris, S. H., 3
Fisman, K., 3, 5
Flower, A., 5, 90, 97
Freeman, M., 53
Freeman, T., 97

G

Gathercole, C., 97
Gee, J. P., 17, 19, 20, 21, 34
Gergen, K., 121
Gergen, M., 121
Glaser, S., 61
Goldstein, K., 96
Gordon, S., 95, 102
Grudin, R., 11, 89

H

Hamilton, H., 1, 6, 10, 120
Haynes, S., 5, 90, 97
Heir, D., 5
Helm-Estabrooks, T., 5
Heritage, J., 21, 22, 24, 25, 26
Hollingworth, H., 17
Hood, L., 58
Hunt, M., 90
Hutchinson, J., 56, 58, 60, 69

I

Irigaray, L., 4

J

Jackson, J., 90, 91, 97, 111
Jefferson, G., 22, 64, 70, 71
Jensen, M., 56, 58, 60, 69
Johnstone, B., 96
Jorgensen, J., 121

K

Kasniak, A., 97
Katzman, R., 3
Keenan, E., 96
Kelly, L., 90, 91, 97, 104
Kelly, M., 3
Kempler, D., 90
Keretz, A., 3, 5
Kintsch, W., 18
Kirshner, H., 3
Kraeplin, E., 2

L

Labov, W., 20
Landauer, T., 124
Lebowitz, B. D., 3
Lerner, G. H., 27
Light, E., 3
Linde, C., 13, 104
Linton, M., 11, 13, 130
Lubinski, R., 10, 116, 117, 118, 119

M

Maier, S., 117
Mandelbaum, J., 21, 22, 23, 85, 86
Marshall, V., 124
Martin, A., 4
Martin, O., 3
McLaughlin, M., 61
McMohan, A., 124
Meacham, J., 14, 15
Merriam, S., 124
Miller, I., 119
Mishler, E., 1, 8, 9, 21, 64, 84, 116
Mullin, J., 125
Myers, F., 9

N

Neisser, U., 13
Nicholas, M., 5
Nofsinger, R., 22, 23, 24, 25, 26, 42, 76
Norman, D., 17, 18
Norman, W., 119
North, A., 5, 90, 97

O

Obler, L., 5
Ochs, E., 96

P

Pearlin, L., 125
Peterson, C., 117
Pincus, A., 124
Pirozzolo, F., 67
Polkinghorne, D., 12
Prizzolo, F., 3

R

Radley, A., 12
Ramanathan, V., 1, 2, 97, 104
Reisberg, B., 3
Revere, V., 124
Rhudick, P., 124
Riley, K., 124
Ripich, D., 5
Rocisano, L., 58
Ross, M., 13
Rumelhart, D., 90
Rutter, M., 97

S

Sabat, S., 2, 5, 6
Sacks, H., 22, 63, 71, 72, 84
Saffran, E., 3
Schafer, D., 124, 125
Schank, R., 16, 91
Schegloff, E. A., 25, 63, 71, 72
Schneck, M. K., 3
Schouten, T., 90, 91, 97, 111
Schwartz, M, 3
Seligman, M., 117
Sherman, E., 11, 12
Srull, T. K., 95, 103

Steir, F., 121
Strauss, C., 9, 90, 96, 98, 102, 132
Stubbs, M., 7, 132
Swihart, A., 3, 67, 132

T

Tannen, D., 96, 97, 117
Tarman, V., 124
Terrell, B., 5
Tobin, S., 124
Tomoeda, C. K., 4, 97
Tonkin, E., 11
Tracy, K., 103
Tulving, E., 17, 18

U

Ulatowska, H., 5, 90, 97

V

Villaume, W., 90, 91, 97, 111

W

Waletzky, J., 20
Watson, L., 7
Watson-Franke, M. B., 7
Webb, W., 3
Weisser, S., 11
Wells, C., 3
Whitaker, H., 96
Whitlatch, C., 125
Wiemann, J., 61
Wyer, R. S., 95, 102, 103

Z

Zarit, S., 125

Subject Index

A

Adjacency pairs, 22
Affirmations, 42–45
Aging process, 12
Alzheimer's disease
  and central nervous system, 56
  background of, 2–3
  diagnosis of, 3, 67
  early stages of, 31, 93–110, 117
  inability to narrate, 54
  later stages of, 110–113
  linguistic studies on, 1–2, 5
  patient isolation, 92
  phases of, 3
Anthropologists, cognitive, 9
Anxiety, 3
Assessments, 23
Audiences
  role of, 15–16, 18–19, 71–88, 116, 125–126
  turns of, see Narrative turns
Autism, 97

B

Baby boomers, 3
Boundedness, 90, 95, 98–102, 109, 114
Brain
  information processing of, 90, 94
  of Alzheimer's patients, 3

C

Caregivers
  role of, 116, 118, 125
  training of, 10, 121–125
Case studies
  narratives at day-care centers, 53–70, 91, 100–110, 112–113
  narratives in home setting, 32–44
  narratives with spouse, 71–88, 118
  patient backgrounds, 8, 30–32, 93–94
Chronology of events, 13
Coherence, see Wellformedness
Cohesion, 5
Collaborations in narrative interactions, 27
Communication research, 10
Context, see Environment

Continuity elements, see also Discontinuity elements, 7, 21–28, 52, 74, 119, 123, and environment, 43, 45
  in narratives at home, 40–44
Conversation
  conversation-analysis, 21–22
  pauses in, 63–64
  vs. narration, 53–54, 73–74, 77–78, 87
Conversations With an Alzheimer's Patient (Hamilton), 5

D

Day-care centers, adult, 7, 116
  description of, 31–32, 91–92
  patient–staff interaction in, 92
Dementia, 2–3, 58, 97, 117
Discontinuity elements, see also Continuity elements, 7, 23–24, 28, 61–62, 66–70, 120, 124
  repair utterances, 71–88
Discourse analysis, 2, 10
Disorientation, 3

E

Echolalia, see Repetition
Encoding, 94–95
Environment, 2, 13, 17, 82
  in case studies, 7
  and continuity in speech, 60–61, 66, 69
  distractions in, 58, 70
  effect on recall, 121
  and social interactions, 17, 90, 116
  stimulation in, 5
Ethnographic methods, 8, 30–32, 89, 115
Event schema hierarchy, 102–103
Extended reportability, 13

F

Formulations, 26–27, 41–42, 44–45

G

Gerontology, 10

I

Incontinence, 3, 111

136

Subject Index

Inquiry guided research, 8
Interactions, 22–23
    continuity elements in, 24–29, 40–44
    misalignment in, 64–65, 69
    processes of, 6, 8–9
    with spouse, 71–88, 118
Interventionist strategies, 121–125
Interviews, 1, 4–5, 7–9, 120
Intonation, 32

L

Language deterioration, 2, 4–5
    over time, 90, 110–114
Learned helplessness, 117, 119
Lexical retrieval, 3
Life history
    accuracy of, 13
    and memory processes, 15–19
    analysis of, 6–7
    in late stages of Alzheimer's, 114–115
    repetition in, 90
    schematic analysis of, 104–110
    temporal aspects of, 11–13, 53
Listening skills, 121–123

M

Macroethnographic methods, 8, 115
Meaning-based discourse, *see also* Text-based discourse, 96–98, 108, 110
Memory
    and self-identity, 1, 12
    in late stages of Alzheimer's, 3
    loss of short-term, 67, 94
    painful memories, 12
    processes of, 15–19
    semantic, 114
    "significant memories," 11, 13
Metamessages, 117–118
Microethnographic methods, 8, 115

N

Narrative sequences
    boundedness in, 90, 95, 98–102, 109, 114
    examples of, 33–52, 54–70, 118–119, 121–123
    marking of, 32
Narrative turns, 21–22, 70, 82, 116, 119
    interference of recipient turns, 87
    interviewer delay of, 6
    passing turns, 62
    positioning of, 9
    sequential implicativeness, 22
Newsmarkers, 24–25, 30–41, 44–45

O

Overaccomodation, 84, 88

P

Passivity, 117
Pauses, 32, 120
    dyadic, 60–61, 65–66
    extended, 62–66
    transition-relevant places of, 63
Perseveration, 3, 5–6, 96–97
Personality changes, 3
Pitch contours, 20
Psycholinguistic research, 1–7, 90, 120
Psychology, cognitive, 90

Q

Questions, open-ended, 123

R

Recall, 15, 17, 28
    and interactive wellformedness, 21–24
    and narrative wellformedness,
    and self-reminding, 51–52
    factual, 14
    failures in, 82
    functions of, 29
    interferences in, 19–21, 68
    theory of, 8
Recognition, 17–19, 28, 82, 87, 118
    of family members, 3
    tests for measuring, 17
Reminding, 15–17, 28, 53
    positioning of reminding prompts, 66–70
Reminiscence, 12
    to preserve identity, 124
Remnant skills, 2, 115
Repair, 72–89
    event-oriented, 82–83
    extended turns in, 76
    self-initiated vs. other-initiated, 70–71
    self-repair, 70–71
Repetition, 6, 10, 90, 94, 96, 99, 114

S

Scaffolding, 57, 69

Schemata, 90, 94–96
Schematic analysis, 9–10, 104–110
Schizophrenia, 97
Self-identity, 1, 12, 114–115, 124
Self-narrative, 12–15
Self-reminding
    toward beginning of sequences, 45–48, 68
    toward end of sequences, 48–52, 68
Self-repair, 71–72
Senility, *see* Dementia
Sequential implicativeness, 22
Setting, *see* Environment
Situational cues, 117
Social skills, 61
Spaced-retrieval method, 124
Speaker involvement, 97
Speech
    connected, 39–40, 60–61
    egocentric, 58–60, 70
    lapses in, 57–58, 61–62
    reciprocal nature of, 6
Stanza segmentation, 9, 19–21, 28, 33, 54–55, 59–60, 71–72
Sustainers, 25, 44–45

T

Tests
    Boston Naming Test, 94
    for measuring recognition, 17
    minimental tests, 94
Text-based discourse, *see also* Meaning-based discourse, 91, 97–98, 111
Theoretical framework, 11–29
Tone, 32
Topic shifts, 32, 69
Turn taking, *see* Narrative turns

W

Wellformedness, 6–7, 9
    absence of, 53–70
    in narratives at home, 32–39
    interactive, 21–24, 44–45
    narrative, 19–21
    of life histories, 14